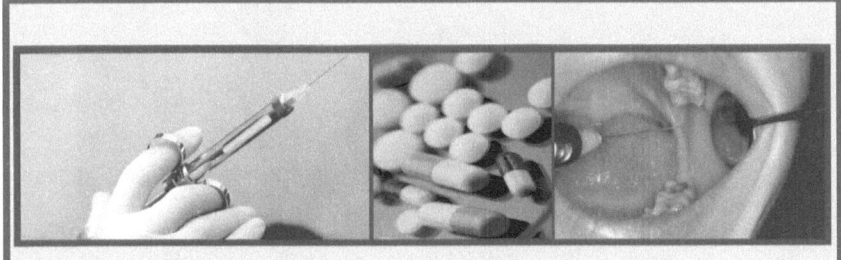

COMPREHENSIVE
PHARMACOLOGY
for Clinical Dentistry

DR. MAAZ.M.AYAZ (BDS)

For book orders, email orders@traffordpublishing.com.sg

Most Trafford Singapore titles are also available at major online book retailers.

Note: Medical knowledge is a constantly changing field. The new researches are taking place throughout the year, therefore, the author and publisher will not be responsible for any harm caused to the patient by the use of these drugs. Practitioners are directed to keep themselves up dated regarding the knowledge of different products provided by the manufacturers.

Printed in Singapore.

ISBN: 978-1-4669-3187-9 (sc)
ISBN: 978-1-4669-3188-6 (hc)
ISBN: 978-1-4669-3189-3 (e)

Trafford rev. 12/19/2012

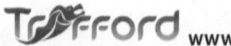 www.traffordpublishing.com.sg
Singapore
toll-free: 800 101 2656 (Singapore)
Fax: 800 101 2656 (Singapore)

This book is dedicated to my beloved father
Engr. Ayaz Mahmood Khan

Patrons:

Iram Abbas
BDS, MCPS, FCPS
Professor and Head of Oral and Maxillofacial Surgery
Department of Dentistry
Ayub Medical College, Abbottabad

Waqar ur Rehman Qureshi
BDS, MSc (UK)
Associate Professor
Oral Dental and Maxillofacial Surgery
Department of Dentistry
Ayub Medical College, Abbottabad

Sumbal Tariq
MBBS, MCPS, FCPS (Med.)
Assistant Professor
Department of Pharmacology & Therapeutics
Ayub Medical College, Abbottabad

Wisal Mahmood Khan
MBBS, MRCS (UK)
Surgical Specialist
Emergency Hospital Scheme, FATA
Pakistan

Asif Waseem
B.Pharm, Pharm.D

TABLE OF CONTENTS

PART I
General Pharmacology

PART II
Therapeutic drug Classifications

PART III
Pharmacology in Dental practice

PREFACE

Students and doctors in the profession of dentistry in developing countries, particularly Pakistan, are aware of the fact that there is no book of Pharmacology exclusively for Dentistry easily available to them. Although there are many books of Dental Pharmacology available in the West, these books are not only difficult to be accessed by the students but are also very expensive. Resultantly, the BDS students make use of books meant for MBBS and explore these—sometimes enormous and always expensive—books for Drugs required in Dentistry. The practice, therefore, seemed to me quite time-consuming and expensive during my BDS studies.

I had conceived the idea of a book of Pharmacology exclusively meant for dentistry. After my graduation, the idea had nourished which led me to compile such notes in the form of a book of pharmacology for dentistry that could be used by BDS professionals without consulting and combing books of MBBS.

I, therefore, compiled this book. I may pertinently mention here that the book is a mere compilation of notes, copied verbatim, from various authentic books authored by reputed authors of the world. I have not added anything significant from my own knowledge or opinion. Key to References has been given at the end of the book.

The book describes the drugs commonly used in dental practice, and is a sincere effort on my part to help BDS students get rid of scavenging various books of MBBS and to save time. Perhaps, mature authors and readers may even get annoyed on my work. However, I believe that—keeping in mind the needs of BDS students and beginners in the field of dentistry—my endeavour shall certainly be useful. Anyhow, the book is before you to judge and to convey your frank comment and opinion for improvement. All mistakes are, of course, mine and the entire credit goes to those authors I have consulted and taken notes from.

In this compilation, I am earnestly indebted to my teachers, Mrs. Iram Abbas, Mr. Waqar ur Rehman, and Ms. Sumbal tariq who encouraged me to venture into this small but vital project and helped me regularly by extracting time from there busy schedule. My thanks are also due to my uncle, Dr. Wisal Mahmood Khan (MRCS, UK), whom I have been always pestering to check and edit different parts of the book.

Maaz Mahmood Ayaz, BDS
Abbotabad, 2012

ABOUT THE BOOK

COMPREHENSIVE PHARMACOLOGY for Clinical Dentistry is a unique collection of therapeutic drugs relevant to dentistry. It has the following salient features.

It consists of three parts.

- Part I is an "Introduction to pharmacology" that contains necessary information regarding General Pharmacology important for dental students.
- Part II is a "Therapeutic Drugs Classification" that contains Classes of Drugs, which are important for dental students and dental practitioners. Special feature of 'Dental consideration' has been added at the end of most chapters so, that dental students must know how to deal with a patient using that particular drug, during dental procedures in his office. Mechanism and mode of actions have been kept short and simple for dental students. In some chapters, 'Dental uses' have been highlighted separately under the heading of 'Indications' in addition to medical uses. In the side effects, only those side effects are mentioned that are most significant and important from dental point of view. In the 'Individual drugs', only those drugs are mentioned, which are commonly

used in clinical practice in our region and important form dental point of view.

- Part III is "Pharmacology in Dental Practice", contains information regarding Drugs that are directly used by Dentist in his office.

ABBREVIATIONS

ACTH	adrenocorticotrophic hormone
ADP	adinosine diphosphate
AF	atrial fibrillation
AIDS	acquired immuno deficiency syndrome
AMP-kinase	adenosine monophosphate kinase
Approx.	approximately
b.i.d	two times per day
BP	blood pressure
BPH	benign prostate hypertrophy
Ci$^-$	chloride ion
cAMP	cyclic Adenosine monophosphate
CHF	chronic Heart failure
CMV	cytomegalo Virus
CNS	central nervous system
COPD	chronic obstructive pulmonary disease
CSF	cerebrospinal fluid
CV	cerebrovascular
CVA	cerebrovascular accident
CVS	cardiovascular system
CYP	cytochrome P 450 [system]
DIC	disseminated intravascular coagulation
e-g	for example

EGF	epidermal growth factor
FEIBA	factor eight inhibitory bypassing activity
FFP	fresh Frozen plasma
FSH	follicle stimulating hormone
GABA	gamma amino butyric acid
GI	gastro-intestinal
GLUT-4	glucose transport 4
GMP	guanosine monophosphate
GU	gastro-urinary
HF	heart failure
Hg	mercury
HIV	human immuno deficiency virus
Hrs	hours
HSV	herpes simplex virus
IM	intra-muscular
INR	international normalized ratio
IP3	inositol triphosphate
IV	intra-venous
Kg	kilogram
L.A	local anaesthesia
LMWHs	low molecular weight heparins
LTC4	leukotriene C 4
MAO	monoamine oxidase
MFPDs	myofacial pain dysfunction syndrome
mg	milligram
MHC	major histocompatibility complex
MI	myocardial infarction
ml	millilitre
mm of Hg	milllimeter of mercury
mRNA	messenger RNA
MRSA	methicillin resistance staphylococcus aureus
Na^+	Sodium ion
NADPH	nicotinamide adenine dinucleotide phosphate
NADPH-P450	nicotinamide adenine dinucleotide phosphate-P 450

NIDD	non insulin dependant diabetes mellitus
nMol	nano mole
NPH	insulin Isophane insulin
NSAIDs	non-steroidal anti-inflammatory drugs
O.D	once daily
OTC	over the counter (drugs)
PABA	para-aminobenzoic acid
PBP	penicillin binding protein
PDGF	platelet-dependant growth factor
PG d2	prostaglandin D-2
PG G2	prostaglandin G-2
PMR	polymyalgia rheumatica
PPAR	peroxisome proliferator—activated receptor
PT	prothrombin time
PTT	partial thromboplastin time
q.i.d	four times daily
RAS	recurrent aphthous stomatitis
RCT	root canal treatment
SC	sub-cutaneous
SDD	sub-therapeutic dose doxycycline
SER	smooth endoplasmic reticulum
S/L	sub-lingual
SSRIs	selective serotonin reuptake inhibitors
STX	saxitoxin
t.i.d	three times a day
TMJ	temporo mandibular joint
TNF	tumor necrosis factor
TSH	thyroid stimulating hormone
TTX	tetrodotoxin
TXA2	thromboaxane A2
UDPGA	uridine diphosphate glucuronic acid
V_D	volume of distribution
VWF	von-willibrand factor
VZV	varicella zoster virus

PART I

General Pharmacology

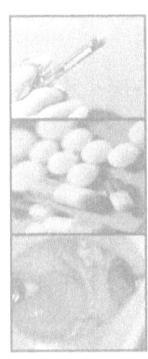

CHAPTER 1

Introduction to Pharmacology

WHAT IS PHARMACOLOGY?

It is the science of properties of drugs and their effects on the body. It is one of the biomedical disciplines but its boundaries are not sharply defined nor are they constant. In this discipline, we understand what drugs do to living organisms, and in particularly how their effects can be applied to therapeutics.

Other related subjects to pharmacology are:

Biotechnology: It constitutes the production of drugs or other useful products by biological means (such as production of antibiotics from microorganisms or production of monoclonal antibodies)

Pharmacogenetics: It includes the genetic influence on response to drugs like familial idiosyncratic reaction (an unusual and unexpected sensitivity exhibited to a particular drug such that a standard dose causes an excessive effect) that occurs in few individuals while other individuals are completely free from such reaction. Other inherited disorder that influences response to drugs is; For example, glucose-6-phosphatase deficiency, a sex linked disorder in which an affected individual may have haemolysis if exposed to certain drugs e-g antimalarial drug (primaquine).

Pharmacogenomics: it involves the use of genetic information to guide the choice of drug therapy on an individual basis.

Pharmacoepidemiology: it is the study of drug effects at a population level. It is concerned with the variablility of drug effects between individuals in a population. So they are constantly watched by regulatory authorities whether to license a new drug for therapeutic purpose or not.

Difference between drug and medicine:

Drug can be defined as a chemical substance of known structure, other than a nutrient or an essential dietary ingredient, which when administered to a living organism, produces a biological effect.

Drugs may be synthetic chemicals, chemicals obtained from plants or animals, or biogenetically manufactured.

Medicine, on the other hand, is a chemical preparation that usually contains one or more drugs so that when administered it produces a therapeutic beneficial effect.[1]

ROUTES OF ADMINISTRATION OF DRUGS:

There are many routes of drug administrations depending upon the properties of drugs and the need for therapeutic requirement.

We have two types of drug administrations.

1. Enteral:

When the drug is given by mouth, it is known as enteral drug administration. It has further two types:

a. Oral
b. S\L

a. <u>Oral</u>: it is the easiest way of self-drug administration and has minimal or no systemic infection involvement.

When drug is administered by oral route, it undergoes absorption from GIT. Hence, the drug is exposed to harsh GI environment. The site of absorption is duodenum however stomach can also act as a site of absorption. As the drug is absorbed into the circulation it undergoes first pass effect (hepatic circulation) after which it enters into systemic circulation.

Because of first pass effect the amount of drug reaching the target site is reduced therefore, we give the drug in sufficient amount in order to reach the target site.

b. <u>Sublingual</u>: the drug is placed under the tongue and it is then absorbed into systemic circulation directly, by-passing the harsh environment of GIT and first pass-effect. The advantages include rapid absorption, rapid onset of action, low incidence of infection and convenience administration.

2. Parenteral:

It involves the administration of drug directly across body's defence barrier into the systemic circulation.

Indications include when the drug is poorly absorbed from GIT or when the drug is subject to harsh GI environment. In addition it is also use for unconscious patient.

It has further three main types.

a. IV
b. SC
c. IM

a. Intravenous: In this route the drug is injected directly in to the systemic circulation (veins) thus by-passing harsh GI environment and first pass effect. It is used for drugs that are not absorbed from GI track. Disadvantages include, the drug cannot be reversed by emesis, the chance of infection is high, it may cause hemolysis and other adverse reactions like allergic reactions or harm due to too rapid administration.

b. Subcutaneous: This route of drug administration requires absorption from the site of injection. The drug is injected into the subcutaneous tissue from where it is absorbed slowly in to the circulation. The absorption is further slowed down by adjunctive use of epinephrine. Epinephrine is vasoconstrictor which limits the drug concentration to the site of injection. Commonest example is that of local anaesthetic (e-g Lidocaine) which is administered along with epinephrine. (see chapter36 on Local anaesthetics)

c. Intramuscular: This route of drug also requires absorption from the site of injection. The drug is injected into the muscle in either an aqueous solution or specialized depot preparation. From the aqueous solution, absorption is fast whereas from depot preparation it is slow. The vehicle used is non-aqueous suspension of *polyethylene glycol*. As the vehicle gets diffuse out of the site, the drug becomes concentrated at the site of injection from where it is absorbed slowly into circulation over a prolonged period.

Other routes:

Inhalational: In this route, the drug is delivered rapidly across the large surface area of respiratory epithelium.

It is most potent for the patients with respiratory complaints (e-g asthma, COPD) as the drug is administered locally to the site. Examples include inhalation of Corticosteroids, albuterol and Salbutamol (beta-agonists).

Intranasal: in this route the drug is absorbed through the nasal mucosa in to the circulation. It is commonly used for patients with upper respiratory problems (e-g allergic rhinitis). Examples include, corticosteroids (Beclometasone, mamotesone), and other nasal decongestants (oxymetazolin, xylometazoline and pseudoephedrine).

Topical: In this, the drug is applied topically to mucosa (e-g oral mucosa) to achieve maximum local effects. Examples include topical use of antifungal drugs (clotrimazoles), corticosteroids for RAS.

Transdermal: In this, the drug is applied locally on the skin site where local effect of drug is desired. Examples include use of transdermal patch of Nitroglycerin for angina, contraceptive patch once-a-week for contraception.

This route is used mostly for sustained release of drug.

Rectal: In this, the drug is placed locally into the rectum from where it is absorbed into the circulation. This route is used when the patient is unable to take oral medication or if the patient is vomiting. Example includes placement of diazepam in children with status epilepticus.[2]

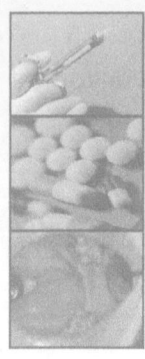

CHAPTER 2
Pharmacokinetics

DEFINITION:

It is the study of measure of how drug concentration in the body changes with time. It includes absorption, distribution, metabolism and excretion.

ABSORPTION:

Absorption is the transfer of drug from its site of administration to the blood stream.

The rate and efficiency of absorption depends upon the route of administration. For example, if the route of administration is IV then the absorption is complete that is the complete drug has accessed to the blood stream.

On the other hand if the route of administration is oral then partial absorption may take place, that is the drug will first be dissolved in GI fluid then the presence of food may also affect the drug absorption and finally it enters into the blood stream via intestinal epithelial mucosa.

Bioavailability:

Bioavailability is the fraction of administered drug that reaches the systemic circulation. Which means the proportion of a drug that is delivered to a site of action in the body. This is usually the amount entering the circulation and may be low when the drugs are given by mouth. It is expressed as the fraction of drug that gains access to the systemic circulation in a chemically unchanged form.[2]

Factors affecting bioavailability:

1) First-pass effect: when the drug is administered orally it is absorbed into the hepatic circulation after which the drug is metabolised in the liver, So the amount of unchanged drug that accesses the systemic circulation is decreased. Examples include the metabolism of Lidocaine and propanolol which undergoes heavy metabolism in the liver.

2) Chemical instability: there are some drugs which are chemically unstable in GI pH; for example, Penicillin G.

3) Drug solubility: majority of the drugs are either weak bases or weak acids because neither too hydrophilic drug can pass through rich lipid bi-layer membrane nor too hydrophobic drugs can pass, as they are very unstable in aqueous medium outside cell membrane.

4) Drug Formulation: the ease of solubility and the rate of absorption is influenced by drug formulation like, enteric coatings, salt form, crystal polymorphism and particle size.[2]

DISTRIBUTION:

Volume of distribution: V_D

It is a hypothetical volume of body fluid into which a drug is dispersed. Or it is the volume of plasma that would contain the total body content of the drug at a concentration equal to that in the plasma.

Water compartments of body:

Plasma (5% of body weight)
Interstitial fluid 16%
Intracellular fluid 35%
Transcellular fluid 2%
Fat 20%

Lipid soluble drugs reach all compartments and may reach fats as well.

Lipid insoluble drugs donot go out of interstitial fluid. They do remain in plasma and interstitial fluid.

Therefore, the volume of distribution becomes more than total body fluid when the drugs accumulate outside the plasma compartment (like fats).

Blood-brain barrier:

It consists of continuous layer of endothelial cells joined by tight-junctions and surrounded by pericytes. By the virtue of this blood-brain barrier, brain remains inaccessible to many drugs including lipid soluble drugs. However, when there is inflammation (e-g meningitis) this barrier is disrupted so, some drugs may pass into the brain. The example of this is Penicillin given intravenously in severe meningitis instead of administering intrathecally.

The blood-brain barrier remains a barrier in normal circumstances. For example, Methylnaltrexone bromide is a mu-receptor opioid antagonist, which does not cross blood-brain barrier so its action remains unaffected.

Drugs limited to plasma compartment:

Some drugs are confined to only plasma by the virtue of their molecular size. Example includes *Heparin* drug which has a larger molecular size and cannot leak out through the capillaries.

Another cause for the drug concentration limited to plasma is the ability of a drug to bind to plasma albumin. As the drug exert its pharmacological effect when it enters into the interstitial fluid, in order to meet this demand repeated doses of drug is administered so that all the drug molecules saturate the plasma proteins and the excess one escapes into the interstitial fluid.

This gives rise to a new term *"Loading Dose"*.

So, the Loading dose of a drug can be injected as a single dose to achieve the desired plasma level rapidly followed by an infusion to maintain the steady state (Maintenance dose).

Drugs accessed to Extracellular compartment:

The example of such drugs is *Gentamicin and Vecuronium.*

Because of their low lipid solubility they cannot enter into cell. They also cannot traverse the blood-brain barrier and the placental barrier easily.

Drugs distributed throughout the body water:

Drugs like *phenytoin, ethanol, morphine and tricyclic anti-depressants* are highly lipid soluble so that they can easily enter into the cells therefore, the volume of distribution of these drugs become greater than the total body water. Such drugs are difficult to be removed from the body by haemodialysis, so there overdose management becomes inoperable.[1]

METABOLISM:

Metabolism is one of the processes of drug elimination from the body in addition to excretion.

It consists of catabolism and anabolism, phase 1 and phase 2 reactions.

Phase 1 reaction:

It is a catabolic reaction in which, the products formed may be more toxic and chemically reactive than the parent compound. It includes the incorporation of a reactive group to the drug compound (like—hydroxyl group) this is known as *functionalisation*.

This addition of reactive group then acts as a site for the conjugation process in *phase 2 reaction*.

The phase 1 reaction occurs mainly in the liver, in which enzymes system CYP participates.

CYP enzymes are basically haem proteins, they are present in SER of liver cells which gets disintegrate and release these enzymes.

There are seventy four CYP gene families amongst which only CYP1, CYP2 and CYP3 are used in drugs metabolism in human liver. These enzymes have differences in their amino acid sequence.

The net result of phase 1 reaction is addition of oxygen atom to the drug molecule to form a hydroxyl group.

This phase 1 reaction requires the presence of a drug (substrate), cytochrome P450 enzyme, NADPH, molecular oxygen and flavoprotein (NADPH-P450 reductase).

Drugs that act as a substrate for this P450 enzyme system are; Alcohol, caffeine, Codeine, cyclophasphamide, Ibuprofen, indinavir, nifedipine, omeprazole, Paracetamol, phenytoin, repaglinide and Tolbutamide.

Phase 2 reaction:

They are anabolic and it involves conjugation of drug molecule after phase 1 reaction or directly on parent drug.

They also take place in the liver. The resultant products are inactive with some exceptions. For example, morphine is converted into active metabolite known as morphine 6-glucoronide, which acts as an analgesic. Glucoronide formation occurs which involves the production of uridine diphosphate glucoronic acid (UDPGA), from which glucoronic acid is transferred to electron rich atom on the substrate (drug) to form an ester, amide or thiol bond.

Active metabolites of some drugs:

Drugs	Active metabolites
Azathioprine	Mercaptopurine
Prednisone	Prednisolone
Cortisone	Hydrocortisone
Enalapril	Enalaprilat
Zidovudine	Zidovudine trisphosphate
Morphine	Morpine 6-glucoronide
Diazepam	Nordiazepam

Toxic metabolites of some drugs:

Drugs	Toxic Metabolites
Diazepam	Oxazepam (toxic)
Paracetamol	N-Acetyl-p-benzoquinone imine

CYP 450-enzyme inhibition:

Some drugs inhibit CYP 450 enzyme by competitive inhibition, for example quinidine (an antimalarial drug).

While some drugs inhibit enzyme by non-competitive inhibition for example, ketoconazole.

As a result, of these inhibitions many clinically important drug-drug interactions take place.

CYP 450-enzyme induction:

Many drugs induce this enzyme leading to increased drug toxicity and carcinogenicity.

For example, paracetamol is metabolised to toxic metabolite known as N-Acetyl-p-benzoquinone imine. So, if other drugs which induce this enzyme used concomitantly with paracetamol, they will increase the toxicity of paracetamol in human body.

Drugs that induce microsomal enzymes include *carbamazepine, ethanol and rifampicin*. They increase the oxidation and conjugation processes when administered repeatedly.

EXCRETION:

Drugs and metabolites renal excretion:

Some drugs are excreted very fast such as penicillin, while other drugs are excreted very slowly from the kidney like Diazepam. The rest falls in between these two extremes.

Renal drug excretion mainly includes three processes:

1. Glomerular filtration:

Those drugs that have molecular weight less than 20,000 can readily pass glomerular capillaries. Plasma albumin has molecular weight of about 68,000 therefore any drug, which binds to plasma albumin, will not be filtrated through glomerular capillaries.

For example, Warfarin drug is 98% bound to plasma albumin, only 2% of the drug will be excreted via kidney. Therefore, its clearance by glomerular filtration is quite reduced.

2. Tubular secretion:

Most of the drug molecules remain in the peritubular capillaries and only a small amount is filtered via glomerular filtration. So the drugs from peritubular capillaries are transported into the tubular lumen by two carrier systems. a) OAT and b) OCT. a) OAT carrier transports drug molecules against electrochemical gradient and transport acidic drugs, where as b) OAT carrier transports drug molecules down an electrochemical gradient and transports basic drugs.

Hence, those drugs, which are bound to plasma albumin (which cannot be filtrated by glomerulas filtration), are transported by carrier-mediated system therefore their clearance is maximal from the plasma. For example, penicillin is bound to plasma albumin by 80%; it is cleared almost completely by proximal tubule secretion.

Drugs transported by OAT carrier system:

Furosemide
Penicillin
Indomatacin
Thiazide diuretics

Drugs transported by OCT carrier system:

Morphine
Pethidine
Quinine

3. Diffusion across the renal tubule:

99% of water of the filtrate is reabsorbed from the tubule, with remaining 1% in the tubules. *Lipid soluble drugs* are poorly excreted, while *polar drugs* (as they have low permeability in tubules) remain in the lumen and excreted in much quantity.

Examples of polar drugs are *Digoxin* and *aminoglycosides antibiotics.*

Therefore care must be taken on administering these drugs if the patient has renal function impairment and/or elderly patients.[1]

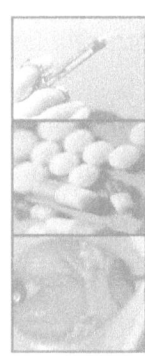

CHAPTER 3

Interaction of Drugs with Receptors

In pharmacology, receptor is considered to be a biological molecule to which ligand (a drug) binds and produces intracellular response. This response is biophysical and /or biochemical activity of the cell. A cell has many types of receptors, and each receptor is receptive for a particular kind of drug. When a drug gets bind to receptor, drug-receptor complex is formed which ultimately produces a biological effect with the help of a messenger, messenger may be hormones, transmitters or other mediators.

For the sake of simplicity, we have classified receptors into different kinds, namely:

1. G-protein coupled receptors
2. Ligand-gated ion channels intracellular receptors enzyme-linked receptors
3. Intracellular receptors
4. Enzyme-linked receptors

1. G-protein coupled receptors:

They are also known as 7-transmembrane or hepta-helical receptor. They comprise of single peptide that has seven membrane—spanning regions, which are linked to intracellular system via G—protein.

Second messenger, for example, cAMP is activated which does phosphorylation of proteins inside the cell. Receptors for this family include muscarinic acetyl-choline receptor (for cholinergic transmission) and adrenoceptors (alpha and beta receptors).

2. Ligand-gated ion channels:

They are also known as ionotropic receptors. On these receptors fast neurotransmitters act and produce an alteration in flow of ions across cell membrane. Examples include nicotinic acetylcholine receptor and GABA receptor (on which benzodiazepine class of drugs act).

Stimulation of nicotinic receptor results in sodium influx, and generation of action potential ultimately contraction of skeletal muscles.

While stimulation of GABA receptor results in increase chloride influx and hyperpolarization of the cell. (Note: GABA is the main inhibitory neurotransmitter in the CNS, stimulation of which will cause hyperpolarization, which means difficulty in depolarization and decreasing excitability of neurones in CNS.

3. Intra-cellular receptors:

They are also known as nuclear receptors. As both names indicate that, the receptor is mainly present inside the cell, which ultimately acts on nucleus of a cell for gene transcription.

This requires drug to be lipid soluble in order to diffuse into the cell and interact with the receptors. Examples include receptors for steroid hormones, thyroid hormones retinoic acid and vitamin D. As the drug finally reaches nucleus and perform its job their so, its response requires more time to be effective. Cellular responses involve gene expression and protein synthesis which require longer duration for its action approximately thirty minutes or more.

4. Enzyme-linked receptors:

They are also known as kinase-linked receptors as the name indicates most common enzyme-linked receptors have tyrosine—kinase based activity which acts on cytosolic enzyme to produce an activity.

The ligand (drug) binds to extracellular receptor, which induces conformational changes in the domain receptor converting it from inactive to active kinase form. Examples include receptors for insulin, when insulin binds to its receptor the intrinsic tyrosine kinase activity causes autophosphorylation of receptor itself (conformational changes).

This phosphorylated receptor phosphorylates target molecules resulting in the activation of other cellular signals (for example, IP3).

Other examples include platelet derived growth factor PDGF and EGF).[1]

VOLTAGE GATED CHANNELS:

These are ion-channels like that of ligand-gated channels but they are not classified as receptors. These channels open when the cell membrane is depolarized. They include sodium, potassium and Calcium ion channels.

Among them sodium channels are important for the action of local anaesthetics which are frequently used in dentistry.

On sodium channels, Tetrodotoxin, saxitoxin and local anesthetics act causing them to hyperpolarize and making depolarization difficult thus, nerve transmission is blocked producing local anaesthetic effects.

So, we have classified local anaesthetic substances in to different classes based on their biological site and mode of action.

Classification	Definition	Chemical substance
Class A	Those agents which act on the receptor site on the external surface of nerve membrane	Biotoxin for example; tetrodotoxin (TTX), saxitoxin (STX)
Class B	Those agents which act on the receptor site on the internal surface of nerve membrane	Scorpion venom
Class C	Those agents which act by a receptor independent physicochemical mechanism	Benzocaine
Class D	Those agents which act by combination of receptor and receptor independent mechanisms	Lidocaine, Articaine, Mepivacaine and prilocaine [5]

WHAT IS A THERAPEUTIC INDEX?

Therapeutic index is the ratio of dose that produces toxicity to the dose that produces a clinically desired or effective response in a population of individuals.

Therapeutic index = TD_{50}/ED_{50}

TD_{50} is a drug dose that produces a toxic effect in half of the population.

ED_{50} is a drug dose that produces a desired response in half of the population.[2]

PART II

Therapeutic drug Classifications

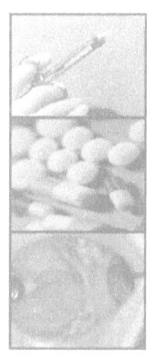

CHAPTER 4

Sympathomimetics

Sympathomimetics are those drugs, which act on adrenergic receptors and activate them or Sympathomimetics are those drugs, which mimic the action of epinephrine or nor-epinephrine.

CLASSIFICATION

This classification is based on the mode of action:

1.   Direct acting:
        Epinephrine
        Norepinephrine
        Levonordefrin
        Isoproterenol
        Dopamine
        Methoxamine
        Phenylephrine

2.   Indirect acting:
      Tyramine
      Amphetamine

Methamphetamine

Hydroxyamphetamine

3. Mixed acting:
    Metaraminol
    Ephedrine

MODE OF ACTION:

Direct acting drugs act by binding directly to adrenergic receptors (alpha and beta) thus stimulating sympathomimetic activity.

Indirect acting drugs act by releasing nor-epinephrine from stores at nerve endings.

Mixed acting drugs act by both above-mentioned type of actions.[10]

Classification based on the type of receptors:

1. Alpha receptors:

    a) Alpha 1 receptor:
        Phenylephrine
        Metaraminol
        Methoxamine
    b) Alpha 1 and Alpha 2:
        Adrenaline
        Noradrenaline

2. Beta receptors:

    a) Beta 1 receptor:
        Prenalterol
        Dobutamine
    b) Beta 2 receptor:
        Salbutamol
        Terbutaline

    c) Beta 1 and Beta 2 receptors:
        Adrenaline
        Isoproterenol

3. Both Alpha and beta receptors:

    Adrenaline
    Dobutamine
    Ephedrine
    Amphetamine

General effects of the adrenergic receptors:

Alpha-1 receptors:

They cause Vasoconstriction, constriction of pupil, contraction of splenic capsule and contraction of trigone-muscle of the urinary bladder.

Alpha-2 receptors:

They produce decrease tone, motility and secretion of GI system. They also decrease insulin secretion.

Beta-1 receptors:

They increase heart rate (positive chronotropic effect), increase heart contractility (positive inotropic effect), increase cardiac output and arrhythmias. They also increase lipolysis.

Beta-2 receptors:

They cause bronchodilation, increase peripheral vasodilation, decrease tone, motility and secretory activity of GI track and increase renin secretion.

Systemic effects of adrenergic agonists: (Particular to epinephrine)
• Cardiovascular system: + Heart rate, ++ stroke volume, +++ cardiac output, ++++ Arrhythmias, ++ coronary blood flow.
• Blood pressure: +++ Systolic arterial, + mean arterial, +,0, diastolic arterial.
• Peripheral circulation: + Cerebral blood flow, +++ splanchnic blood flow.
• Respiratory system: +++ bronchodilation.
• Genitourinary system: —nil—
• Skeletal system: +++ muscle blood flow.
• Metabolic effects: ++ oxygen consumption, +++ blood glucose, +++ blood lactic acid. [5]

INDICATIONS:

See section on Individual Drugs below.

SIDE EFFECTS:

See section on Individual Drugs below.

Contraindications:

Tachycardia occurs due to arrhythmia, tachycardia or heart block is also caused by digitalis toxicity. [5]

Cautions:

Use with caution in hyperthoiridism, diabetes, CHF, cardiac dysarrhythmias, ischemic heart diseases, angina, seizures and history of stroke.

INDIVIDUAL DRUGS:

1. Epinephrine: (Adrenalin)

Pharmacokinetics:

- It can not be given orally because it is destroyed in GI track.
- It is administered subcutaneously or intramuscularly.
- Intravenous injection may cause ventricular fibrillation and therefore is highly dangerous.

Indications:

- For management of acute allergic reactions like anaphylactic shock. Adrenalin is a physiologic antagonist of histamine. (Note: Adrenalin is the only drug that should be present in dental office in a preloaded form)
- For management of bronchospasm.
- For management of cardiac arrest, it is given as an intracardiac injection.
- As a vasoconstrictor for haemostasis.
- As a vasoconstrictor in local anaesthetics to decrease absorption into cardiovascular system.

- As a vasoconstrictor in local anaesthetics to increase the depth of anaesthesia.
- As a vasoconstrictor in local anaesthetics to increase duration of local anaesthesia.
- To produce mydriasis. (pupil dilation)

Side effects:

- CVS, fatal cardiac arrhythmias, angina, increase in high blood pressure may lead to aortic rupture, cerebral haemorrhage.
- Metabolic, increase in lactic acid lead to metabolic acidosis. Increase in blood sugar level predisposes diabetic patient to hyperglycemia.
- CNS, anxiety, fear, and pallor.
- At injection site; bleeding, urticaria, wheal formation and pain. Repeated injection at same site causes necrosis of tissue due to severe vasoconstriction.

Dosages:

- For Haemostasis, epinephrine is used in concentration of 1:50,000.
- For emergency injection, it is used in concentration of 1:10,000.
- Intra cardiac /IV, 0.1-1 mg repeated every 5 minutes.
- *As an adjunct with local anaesthetics,* for 1:100,000-0.01mg/ml (18 microgram per 1.8ml cartridge); for 1:200,000-0.005mg/ml (9 microgram per 1.8ml cartridge).
- Bronchodilation; 0.3-0.5mg SC, IM every 20 minutes as needed.
- Inhalation; 1 inhalation of 1% solution after 20 minutes or as needed.

2. Levonordefrin:

Use as potent vasoconstrictor with local anesthetic (Mepivacaine) in 1:20,000 dilutions. It is 15% as potent vasopressor as epinephrine.

Mode of action:

It appears to act through direct alpha receptor stimulation (75%) with some beta activity (25%), but to lesser degree than epinephrine.

Side effects and over dose are:

- Hypertension
- Ventricular tachycardia
- Anginal episodes in patients with coronary insufficiency.

Other side effects are the same as epinephrine but to lesser extent.

Dosage:

As it is considered 1/6th potent vasopressor as epinephrine so it is used in higher concentration of 1:20,000. Maximum dose that can be administered in local anesthetics is 1mg per appointment; 20ml of a 1:20,000 (11 cartridges).

The concentration in which it is available has clinically the same effect on local anesthetics as does epinephrine of 1:50,000 or 1:100,000 concentration has.

3. Felypressin:

It is a synthetic analogue of antidueretic hormone vasopressin. It is a **non-sympathomimetic amine** categorized as a vasoconstrictor.

(Note: It has been included in this chapter because of its usage in dental local anaesthesia).

Mode of action:

It act as a direct stimulant of vascular smooth muscle. Its actions appear to be more pronounced on the venous than on the arteriolar microcirculation.

Systemic actions:

<u>Corononary arteries</u>; when administered in higher doses it may impair blood flow through coronary arteries.

<u>Vasculature</u>; in high doses felypressin-induced constriction of cutaneous blood vessels which produces facial pallor.

<u>Central nervous system</u>; it has no effect on adrenergic nerve transmission; so it can **be safely administered to hyperthyroid patients** and to anyone receiving MAO inhibitors or tricyclic antidepressants.

<u>Uterus</u>; it has both antidiuretic and oxytocic effect, the latter contraindicates its use in pregnant women.

Indications:

Used as vasoconstrictor in local anaesthetics to decrease its systemic absorption and increase its depth of anaesthesia.

Side effects laboratory and clinical studies demonstrated wide range of safety for this drug, it is highly tolerated by the tissues into which it is administered. It produces less irritation.

Dosage:

0.03 IU/ml, (3% prilocaine is available in Japan, Germany and other countries but not in USA).

Contraindication to Vasoconstrictor administration:

In general, they fall into three categories;
1. Patients with more significant cardiovascular disease.
2. Patients with certain non-cardiovascular diseases like thyroid dysfunction, diabetes and sulfite sensitivity.
3. Patients receiving MAO inhibitors, tricyclic antidepressants and phenothiazines. [5]

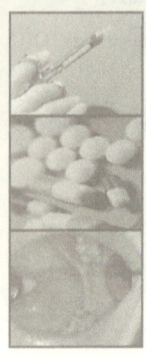

CHAPTER 5

Nasal Decongestants

CLASSIFICATION:

Ephedrine
Pseudoephedrine
Phenylephrine

MODE OF ACTION:

Mostly used decongestants are adrenergic agonists. They act on alpha receptors of arterioles of nasal mucosa causing vasoconstriction thus relieves congestion of nose.

(See also chapter 4 Sympathomimetics)

INDICATIONS:

They are given per oral for nasal blockage due to allergic rhinitis, sinusitis, common cold and other allergies. They are used topically for nasal and nasopharyngeal congestion due to hay fever, allergies and/or sinusitis. They are also used to relieve congestion around

Eustachian tube and relieve ear block and pressure pain during air travel.

ADVERSE EFFECTS:

Topical; nasal dryness, rebound congestion, irritation of nasal mucosa.

Oral; dry mouth and altered taste.

CVS; cardiovascular collapse, tachycardia, arrhythmias, transient hypertension, palpitaion

CNS; anxiety, fear, dizziness, headache, **seizures**, depression [10]

Note: Ephedrine may also cause anorexia and urinary retention in men with prostrate hyperplasia.

INDIVIDUAL DRUGS:

1. **Ephedrine:**

Pharmacokinetics:

- It is well absorbed orally.
- It is 40 % metabolized in the liver.
- Its half life is more than 4 hours.
- It is a poor substrate to MAO
- It is weakly basic and is mostly excreted as such in urine.

Mode of action

It has direct effect on ***alpha, beta 1 and beta 2 receptors*** causing, high blood pressure, bronchodilation and decrease tone, motility and secretion of GI system and nasal decongestion.

Indications:

- It is used as nasal decongestant in patients with hay fever, allergies, sinusitis.
- It is used for bronchospasm due to asthma or COPD.
- It is used for hypotensive shock parenterally.
- It is used in acute hypotension associated with spinal anaesthesia and stokes Adams syndrome with complete heart block.

Side effects:

It may cause excessive hypertension which may result in cerebral hemmorrhage.

Dosage:

Use as 25mg and 50mg capsules for bronchodilation, nasal decongestion and CNS stimulant (25-50mg) every 3-4 hours.

Use as bronchodilator in 12.5-25mg dose subcutaneous, intramuscular and slow intravenous injections.

Use as vasopressor in 25-50mg repeated dose after every 10-15 minutes.

Use as a topical (0.25%) spray for nasal decongestion, 2-3gtt (drops) of solution.

2. **Phenylephrine:**

Dosages:

Intra muscular and Subcutaneous (for mild to moderate hypotension)

It is given in 2-5mg dose which should not exceed initial dose of 5mg Subcutaneously or intramuscularly.

Intravenously it is given in 0.2mg dose with maximum of 0.5mg dose.

For severe hypotension;

10mg IV, use along with 250-500 ml of 5% dextrose and/or 0.9% sodium chloride.

For prophylaxis of hypotension during spinal anaesthesia.

2-3mg IM or SC. 3-4 minutes before spinal anaesthesia is given.

Vasoconstrictor for regional anaesthesia;

Add 1mg to every 20ml of local anaesthesia.

Nasal spray;

2-3gtt (drops) of 0.25% or 0.5% solution into each nostril 3-4 hours as needed.

DENTAL CONSIDERATION:

- Patient may require semi supine position during dental procedure to help with breathing.
- Dryness of mouth may put the patient to caries, periodontitis and candidiasis risk. [10]
- Misuse of nasal sprays may cause severe problem when used for more than 1week or as prescribed by ENT specialist. Problem such as rebound congestion is most common. [10]

SYMPATHOLYTIC DRUGS

They are those drugs, which oppose the effect of sympathetic nervous system. They are divided into three categories.

1) Receptor blocking drugs:
2) Adrenergic neuron blocking drugs:
3) Centrally acting sympatholytics:

Receptor blocking drugs are discussed in detail in the subsequent chapters. Here we will just give the classification of two later categeories

Adrenergic neuron blocking drugs:

Guanethidine
Reserpine
Methyldopa

Centrally acting sympatholytics:

Methyldopa
Reserpine

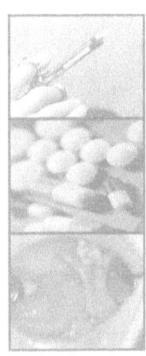

CHAPTER 6

Alpha-adrenergic blocking agents

They fall into the first category "receptor blocking drugs". They are drugs, which prevents stimulation of alpha-adrenergic receptors at the nerve endings of sympathetic nervous system by nor adrenaline and adrenaline.

CLASSIFICATION:

Non-selective (alpha-1 and alpha-2)
    Phenoxybenzamine
    Phentolamine

Selective:
    Alpha-1 blockers:
    Doxazosin
    Prazosin
    Terazosin
    Alfuzosin
    Tamsulosin

    Alpha-2 blockers:
    Yohimbine

MODE OF ACTION:

These drugs block alpha-receptor profoundly affecting blood pressure. They cause blockage of alpha 1—receptors on blood vessels (arterioles and veins) leading to vasodilation which in turns decreases blood pressure. Moreover, Terazosin also causes relaxation of smooth muscles of bladder neck making it useful for BPH. [3]

INDICATIONS:

Foremost it is used for hypertensive patients alone or in combination with other anti hypertensive drugs like beta adrenergic blocker or diuretics. It is useful in older patients for benign prostate hyperplasia (BPH). It is also useful for CHF, and for the management of Reynaud's phenomena.

ADVERSE EFFECTS:

Mouth: Dry mouth may lead to xerostomia.
CVS: palpitation, postural hypotension, arrhythmia
CNS: anxiety, dizziness, decreased libido, depression
Respiratory: nasal congestion, rhinitis, bronchospasm, dyspnea
Miscelleneous: tinnitus, vertigo, headache, lichen planus, pruritus. [10]

Individual drugs:

1. Phenoxybenzamine:

- It is non-selective adrenergic blocking agents for both alpha-1 and alpha-2 receptors.
- Its blockage is irreversible and non-competitive.

Indications:

- o Use for benign prostate hypertrophy.
- o Use for acute hypertensive episodes due to sympathomimetics and MAO Inhibitors or pheochromocytoma.
- o Some times effective in treating Raynaud's disease, fross bite and acrocyanosis.

2. Phentolamine:

- It is non-selective adrenergic blocking agents for both alpha-1 and alpha-2 receptors.
- It blocks alpha-1 and alpha-2 receptors reversibily and competitively.

Indications:

- o Use for vasoconstriction caused by clonidine, Tyramine and MAO inhibitors.
- o It induces reflex cardiac stimulation and is use for left ventricular failure.
- o Use for short term management of pheochromocytoma.
- o It is also use rarely for the treatment of impotence.

3. Doxazosin:

- Peak plasma level is at 2-3 hrs.
- Peak response is by 2-6 hrs.
- Metabolism occurs in liver.
- Due to causing postural hypotension it is not use in 2, 4 or 8 mg initially.

Dosages:

- o For hypertension:
  1mg dose daily, then it can be increase to 2mg and 4mg daily upto 16mg maximum dose depending upon the response of patient's blood pressure.
- o For BPH:
  1mg dose daily then may increase upto 2mg, 4mg and 8mg.

4. Prazosin:

- It is a specific alpha-1 blocker.

Pharmacokinetics:

- o It is given PO.
- o It undergoes first pass effect.
- o Its bioavailability is 50%.
- o It extensively binds to plasma protein.
- o Its half-life is 3-4 hours.

Dosage:

- o 1mg b.i.d or t.i.d, which may be increased upto 6-15mg daily.
- o Paediatric dose (less than 12 yrs of age)
- o Paediatric dose is 0.25-0.5 mg b.i.d or t.i.d adjusted according to response.

DENTAL CONSIDERATION:

- Monitor the vital signs before commencing any dental treatment.
- When changing the position of dental chair from supine to straight, do so, but slowly upright with intervals to avoid syncope.
- As it causes dry mouth so the patient is susceptible to dental caries, periodontal disease and candidiasis.
- Manage dry mouth with tart, sugar free chewing gums (xylitol), or saliva substitute.
- Avoid prescribing mouthwashes containing alcohol (like Listerine)
- Ask patient to avoid using beverages containing caffeine.
- Accomplish fluoride home treatment. [10]

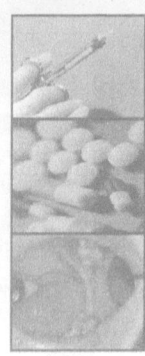

CHAPTER 7

Beta-adrenergic blocking Agents

They fall into first category "receptor blocking drugs". They are drugs, which prevent stimulation of beta-adrenergic receptors at the nerve endings of sympathetic nervous system.

CLASSIFICATION:

Selective beta-1 blockers:
    Acebutalol
    Atenolol
    Esmolol
    Metaprolol
    Bisoprolol

Non-selective beta-1 and beta-2 blockers:
    Propanolol
    Sotalol
    Timolol

Both alpha and beta blockers:
    Labetalol
    Carvedilol

MODE OF ACTION:

They block beta-receptors reversibly.

By blocking beta-1 receptors, they affect heart by decreasing cardiac output, heart rate and AV conduction resulting in overall decrease in blood pressure.

They block the vasodilating effect of catecholomines on peripheral blood vessels leading to vasoconstriction.

They block beta-2 receptors in lungs leading to bronchoconstriction and spasm of bronchioles.

They also decrease production of aqueous humour in eye making it useful for glaucoma patients.

INDICATIONS:

- Use for hypertensive patients alone or in combination with alpha-1 blockers or diuretics.
- Use for angina pectoris, prevention of MI, cardiac arrhythmias and prevention of migraine.
- It is also use more for acute angle glaucoma. [2]

ADVERSE EFFECTS:

Oral: dry mouth (may lead to xerostomia)

CVS: bradycardia, dysarrhythmia, postural hypotension

Respiratory: bronchospasm, dyspnea & wheezing (Contraindicated in asthmatic patients)

GI: diarrhoea, *ischemic colitis, mesenteric arteries thromboses*

Hematologic: *blood dyscrasias, (fever, sore throat and bleeding from gums),* thrombocytopenia (petechia, prura, bleeding)

Allergy: skin rashes, laryngospasm, stridors and anaphylaxis

Sexual dysfunction, (*decrease in libido* in males)

INDIVIDUAL DRUGS:

1. Acebutalol:

Dosages: 400 mg/day (200 mg b.i.d) may increase upto 800 mg per day.

In renal dysfunction, decrease the dose by 50% if creatinine clearance is 50 mL/min/1.73m.square.

Decrease dose by 75% if creatinine clearance is 25mL/min/1.73 m.square.

2. Atenolol:

For hypertension, angina, alcohol withdrawal syndrome, prophylaxis of migraine, ventricular arrhythmias.

Dosages: 50mg dose per day along with other diuretics (thiazide).

Dose may increase upto 100 mg/ day.

3. Propanolol:

Dosages:

For hypertension, 40 mg b.i.d. or 80 mg for sustained release.

For angina, 80-320 mg b.i.d, t.i.d or q.i.d.

For arrhythmias, 10-30 mg t.i.d or q.i.d after meal time and at bed time.

For migraine, 80 mg/day, then increase to 160-240 mg /day. [10]

DENTAL CONSIDERATION:

- If patient is with cardiac problem, consult primary care physician.
- For cardiac patient schedule early morning appointment in order to reduce anxiety of the patient and waiting room time.

- Keep counselling with the patient constantly in order to reduce anxiety.
- While giving local anaesthesia use of epinephrine-free local anaesthetic is beneficial.
- Give local anaesthesia in fully supine position to avoid syncope, then upright the patient slowly to avoid postural hypotension. Ask the patient to keep sitting for at least 2 minutes after supine position.
- Manage dry mouth with tart, sugar free gums, frequent sip of water and/or saliva substitute.
- Advocate fluoride home treatment for caries susceptible patients.
- Manage periodontal diseases with caution.
- Avoid use of epinephrine containing gingival retraction cord.
- Prevent use of alcohol containing mouth rinse.
- Avoid directly dental unit light into eye of glaucoma patient and advise him to wear black glasses during dental treatment.

CHOLINERGIC BLOCKING DRUGS

These drugs block the effect of acetylcholine neurotransmitter on the nerve endings.

They are divided into four groups:

1) *Anti-muscarinic drugs*
2) *Anti-nicotinic drugs*
3) *Ganglion blockings drugs*
4) *Neuromuscular blocking drugs*

For neuromuscular blocking drugs, see chapter 24 skeletal muscle relaxant.

Here we will discuss only anti-muscarinic drugs in the subsequent chapter.

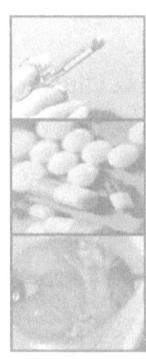

CHAPTER 8

Cholinergic blocking agents

They fall into the first group "Anti-muscarinic drugs".

CLASSIFICATION:

Natural alkaloids:
  Atropine
  Hyoscine

Synthetic alkaloids:
  Benztropine
  Scopolamine (Hyoscine butyl bromide)
  Pirenzepine

MODE AND MECHANISM OF ACTION:

These drugs block cholinergic parasympathetic postganglionic neurons and few sympathetic neurons that are also cholinergic (those neurons that innervate sweat and salivary glands).Atropine in particular competes with acetylcholine for muscarinic receptors. Thus, block its action.

So the parasympathetic activity is blocked while the sympathetic activity remains unaltered.

They have the following effects on different organs.

For example,

1. Eye: they block the muscarinic receptor thus causing persistent mydriasis (dilation of pupil), and cycloplegia (inability to focus for near vision). In patients with narrow angle glaucoma, it causes severe intraocular pressure, so contraindicated in glaucoma patients.

2. GI: they decrease motility of GIT, but donot decrease acid secretion except pirenzepine, which decreases acid secretion on doses that do not antagonize other systems.

3. Urinary bladder: they also decrease motility of bladder so it may be used in children with enuresis (involuntary voiding of urine).

4. *Salivary glands:* they inhibit secretion of salivary glands thus leading to *xerostomia*.

5. Other glands: sweat and lacrimal glands are also affected. When secretion of sweat glands are inhibited this, lead to increase in body temperature. [2]

INDICATIONS:

- Antispasmodic: they decrease the motility of GI track So, Use as an adjunctive with peptic ulcer treatment.
- After the surgery of eye, they are used to cause mydriasis and cycloplegia.
- Treatment of bradycardia, after heart arrest these drugs inhibit parasympathetic activity of heart and cause increase in the heart rate.
- As antidote, they are used as an antidote against poison of irreversible cholinesterase inhibitors (nerve gases poison)

- Pre surgery, they are used to decrease secretion before starting surgery. [2]

ADVERSE EFFECTS:

Mouth: xerostomia
Eye: blurred vision and mydriasis
CNS: confusion
GI: constipation
GU: urinary urgency [10]

INDIVIDUAL DRUGS:

Atropine:

Atropine is a competitive blocking agent as it reversibly blocks the action of acetylcholine at the muscarinic receptor.

Affect of atropine on heart:

It initially causes bradycardia due to cardioinhbitory centre in the medulla.

Affect on circulation:

There is no effect on arterial pressure unless there is hypotension because of bradycardia.

Its large dose causes vasodilation of skin blood vessels. This condition is called atropine-blush.

Indications:

- Use as an adjunctive with peptic ulcer treatment.
- Use for urinary incontinence.
- Use with general anaesthesia in order to decrease salivary and bronchial secretion.

When used parenterally;

- It is use for GI radiography and cardiac dysarrhythmia.

Dosages:
During surgery for drying effect:
Adult's dose is 2 mg.
For anticholinergic effect:
Adults dose is 0.4-0.6 mg (4-6 hours) daily (IM or IV)
For toxicity of cholinesterase inhibitor:
Adult's dose is 2-4 mg IV then followed by 2 mg after every 10 minutes until the muscarinic symptoms disappear and atropine toxicity starts appearing.

As a prophylaxis for excessive respiratory and salivatory secretion or succinylcholine or surgery induced arrhythmias:

Paediatric dose is 0.1 mg for 3 kg, 0.2 mg for 7-9 kg, 0.3 mg for upto 16 kg, 0.4 mg for upto 21 kg, 0.5 mg for upto 31 kg and 0.6 mg for upto 41 kg. [10]

DENTAL CONSIDERATION:

- Monitor the vital signs before commencing any dental treatment.
- Consult patient's primary care physician for having cardiac problem.
- We can use these drugs 20-30 minutes before starting any dental procedure (particular surgery) for drying effect.
- As it causes dryness of eyes so contact lenses of any kind should be removed, moreover the patient should wear black glasses for protection from dental light.
- Give special attention to patients with GI problem or with cardiac arrhythmia.
- Dry mouth effect is for shorter duration so it must not be an issue.

- Advise patient for good oral hygiene maintenance.
- If dry mouth persists after treatment advise patient to take frequent sip of water with meal and chew xylitol chewing gum. [10]

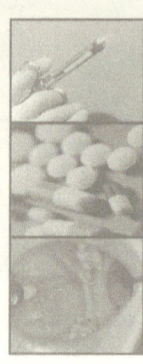

CHAPTER 9

Calcium Channel blocking agents

CLASSIFICATION:

They are divided into two groups:

Dihyropyridines:
    Nifedipine
    Nimodipine
    Nicardipine
    Amlodipine
    Felodipine

Non-Dihyropyridines:
    Verapamil
    Diltiazem
    Bepridil

MODE OF ACTION:

They inhibit the influx of calcium ions through the cell membrane of smooth muscles and cardiac muscles.

On smooth muscles contraction is decreased and relaxation increases leading to vasodilation and ultimately lowering the blood pressure.

On heart contractility of cardiac muscles decreases as well as AV-, conduction also decreases. It also prolongs the repolarization.

As a result, heart oxygen demand is decreased.

Nifedipine: It acts more specifically on vascular smooth muscle than heart muscles.

Nimodipine: It is particularly selective for cerebral blood vessels.

Amlodipine: It is mostly used because it does not weaken the myocardial muscle in left ventricular failure. It is safe in mild to moderate heart failure.

Verapamil: It has more affinity for heart muscle fibres. It causes greater negative inotropic effects than nifedipine but it is a weaker vasodilator.

Diltiazem reduces heart rate although to a lesser extent than verpamil.

Nifedipine and Diltiazem are used in treatment of variant angina caused by spontaneous coronary spasm.

INDICATIONS:

Useful for **hypertension** but high abrupt dose may be avoided because it may lead the patient to heart attack.

It is as useful in lowering blood pressure as ACE inhibitors, but not as effective as ACE inhibitors in preventing kidney failure (as caused by high BP or diabetes).

Use for *prevention of angina* as it decreases heart load.

Use for different heart abnormalities like *cardiac arrhythmias* (AF, paroxysmal ventricular tachycardia) as it decreases heart rate.

Use for the treatment of migraine headache.

Use for the treatment of Reynaud's syndrome.

ADVERSE EFFECTS:

See section on Individual Drugs below.

INDIVIDUAL DRUGS:

1. Nifedipine:

It is mainly an arteriolar vasodilator.

It has minimal effect on heart rate and conduction.

Side effects include flushing, headache, hypotension, peripheral oedema.

Miscellaneous side effects include **constipation**, *gingival hyperplasia* dry mouth, decrease platelet aggregation and *Steven Johnson's syndrome. (Which involves the eyes and skin, target lesion are also seen on skin as seen in erythema multiforme. Rashes on face and trunk of body are common followed by blisters formation). Other causative drugs for Steven Johnson's syndrome are NSAIDS, sulphonamide antibiotics, phenytoin, carbamazepine and allopurinol*

Dosages:

For hypertension: 10-20 mg t.i.d or q.i.d

For angina: 20-30 mg t.i.d or q.i.d

For emergency hypertension: 10-20 mg S/L (capsule is punctured and the contents are squeezed under the tongue). [10]

2. Verapamil:

Adverse effects: gingival hyperplasia, *AV blocks, MI*, CVA and *Steven's Johnson syndrome.*

Dosages:

For hypertension: Dose is from 80 mg three times a day to 360 mg per day.

For angina: Dose is from 80-120 mg t.i.d upto 240-360 mg per day.

DENTAL CONSIDERATION:

- Use anxiety reduction protocol for angina patients.
- We can use anti-anxiety drugs (like diazepam, alprazolam or clonazepam) if anxiety may precipitate angina.
- Monitor vital signs before starting any dental procedure like extraction, RCT or scaling and periodontal surgery.
- Epinephrine containing L.A should be use with caution. Epinephrine dose may not exceed 0.04 mg.
- Consult primary care physician of patient.
- Monitor regularly oral prophylaxis to prevent gingival hyperplasia.

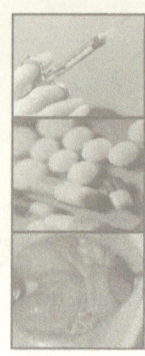

CHAPTER 10

Cardiac glycosides

Glycosides are compounds that are formed by replacing the hydroxyl (-OH) group of a sugar by another group. Glycosides found in plants include some pharmacologically important products (such as digitalis). Other plant glycosides are natural food toxins.

CLASSIFICATION:

Digoxin
Digita lis
Amrinone
Milrinone
Dobutamine [10]

MECHANISM OF ACTION:

These drugs increase the contractility of heart in the following way.

They inhibit the sodium-potassium ATPase in cardiac myocytes. Which in turns increase sodium ions intracellularly, which in turn decreases exchange of Sodium and Calcium ions. Ultimately results in increased intracellular calcium ions that cause forceful contraction of the heart.

Therefore, it is good for systolic HF (Heart failure).

[Note: in systolic HF, There is more stretching of cardiac muscles that cause increase in heart contraction initially, but later due to overstretching of the muscle fibres, the contraction mechanism is diminished causing systolic HF. In contrast, diastolic HF, the heart chambers are unable to relax properly so there is inadequate filling of heart chambers this is diastolic HF. This is common in elderly women.] So glycosides are good for systolic HF, but not for diastolic HF. [2]

INDICATIONS:

- Used for almost all kind of HF, along with ACE-inhibitors and/ or diuretics. (However ACE-inhibitors and diuretics are first choice for mild to moderate HF).
- Also use for patients with atrial flutter and paroxysmal supraventricular tachycardia.

ADVERSE EFFECTS:

Digitalis has *low therapeutic index* (i-e low difference between therapeutic and toxic dose).

Oral: Excessive salivation and sensitive gag reflex.

GI: anorexia, nausea and two stage vomiting (first stage indicates disturbance of GI and gag reflex, second stage indicates stimulation of vomiting centre in brain).

CVS: severe arrythmia

CNS: headache, fatigue, confusion, halos on dark objects and blurred vision. [2]

INDIVIDUAL DRUGS:

Digoxin:

Dosages:
Digitilizing dose (loading dose), 0.4-0.6 mg (4-6 hrs daily)
Maintenance dose, 0.1-0.3 mg (4-6 hrs daily) until desired effect is achieved.
Capsules available: 0.05 mg, 0.1 mg, 0.2 mg

DENTAL CONSIDERATION:

- Follow anxiety reduction protocol for cardiac patients.
- Before the commencement of any dental procedure, consult patient's primary care physician
- Dental radiograph and impression taking may be difficult because of increased sensitivity to gag reflex.
- Excessive salivation may be a hurdle for some dental procedures such as restoration required with composit and RCT.
- Vasoconstrictors in local anaesthesia should be avoided or may be used with high caution.
- Avoid use of gingival retraction cord soaked with epinephrine. [10]

ANTI-HYPERTENSIVE DRUGS

There are many anti hypertensive drugs, initially mild hypertension is treated with a single drug then if hypertension is not controlled adequately second and /or third drug is added to the regimen. (For example, patient started with diuretic is added beta-blockers and vice versa). Third drug may be added such as vasodilator if response is still inadequate. Therapy can be started with ACE-inhibitors or ARBs.

There are certain diseases which restrict the use of some drugs while allow the use of other drugs. (For example in diabetic patients, ACE-inhibitors, Diuretics and ARBs are the choice while for high risk angina pectoris beta-blockers and calcium channel blockers are the drugs of choice).

The aim of antihypertensive drugs is to reduce the risk of complications caused by high blood pressure (Like, cerbrovascular stroke, congestive heart failure, MI, and renal damage).

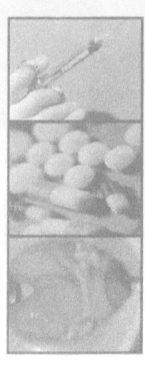

CHAPTER 11
ACE inhibitors

CLASSIFICATION:

Benazepril
Captopril
Enalapril
Fosinopril
Lisinopril
Ramipril

MODE OF ACTION:

ACE-inhibitors as name suggests it blocks the angiotensin converting enzyme So, there is no conversion of angiotensin I to angiotensin II. Angiotensin (II) is a potent vasoconstrictor. Therefore, when it is blocked vasoconstriction activity diminishes and vasodilating activity increases which is further enhanced by increase in level of bradykinin. ACE-inhibitors also decrease the level of aldosterone that in turn decreases salt-water retention.

INDICATIONS:

- Use to treat hypertension (most effectively in white and young).
- Use to decrease the progression of diabetic nephropathy and albuminurea.
- Use to treat chronic heart failure. (compare cardiac glycosides chapter 10)
- Can be start after 24 hrs of MI attack. [2]

ADVERSE EFFECTS:

Oral: dry mouth, ulceration and loss of taste

GI: nausea, vomiting and dry mouth

CVS: hypotension

CNS: sleep disturbance, paraesthesia, headache, dizziness and fatigue.

Miscellaneous: *persistent dry cough,* hyperkalemia, skin rash, angioedema and anaphylaxis

Pregnancy: ACE-inhibitors are fetotoxic and should not be used by pregnant women. [3]

Drug-Drug interaction:

- It causes severe hypotension when use with local anaesthetic as it causes vasodilation and ultimately hypotension.
- Indomatacin: decrease hypotensive effect of ACE-inhibitors.
- NSAIDs: decrease hypotensive effect of ACE-inhibitors
- Antacids: decrease bioavailability of ACE-inhibitors.
- Phenothiazines: increases effect of ACE-inhibitors. [10]

INDIVIDUAL DRUGS:

1. **Captopril:**
   Side effects:
   Erythema multiforme, pemphigus like lesions (bullous pemphigoid), *Steven Johnson syndrome,* pruritus, skin rashes, scalded mouth sensation.
   <u>Oral:</u> Aphthous ulceration, dysgeusia, dries mouth and glossitis.
   <u>Liver:</u> jaundice, hepatitis and cholesistitus.
   <u>Respiratory:</u> bronchospasm, dry cough and dyspnea
   <u>CVS:</u> CHF, *MI*, cardiac arrest
   <u>CNS:</u> *dizziness*
   <u>Hematologic:</u> Aplastic or haemolytic anaemia

   Dosages:
   <u>For hypertension:</u>
   Dose is 25 mg b.i.d or t.i.d, if unsatisfactory response after 1-2 weeks then increases to 50mg b.i.d or t.i.d. it may be increase upto 100-150 mg.
   <u>For heart failure:</u>
   We can start initially with 6.25 mg-12.5 mg t.i.d increase upto 12.5 mg t.i.d, then can increase upto 50mg t.i.d. maximum dose should not exceed 450 mg /day.
   <u>For diabetic nephropathy:</u>
   25 mg t.i.d then increase to 50mg t.i.d.
   <u>For hypertensive crisis:</u>
   S/L 25 mg Captopril is placed.

2. **Enalapril:**
   Side effects:
   See side effects of ACE-Inhibitors.

Dosages:

For hypertension:

5 mg dose per day in two divided doses.

If used along with diuretics then 2.5 mg dose per day is use in daily divided doses.

For emergency:

IV 1.25 mg over 5 minute period, then repeat after every 6 hrs. If patient on diuretics, then 0.625 mg IV, repeat after 1 hour then give 1.25 mg 6 hourly.

DENTAL CONSIDERATION:

- Monitor vital signs at every appointment.
- Asses the risk of cardiovascular events by consultation with the patient's primary care physician.
- Schedule an early morning appointment for dental treatment to reduce waiting room time.
- Give anaesthesia in fully supine position in order to avoid syncope then upright the patient slowly by 2 minutes Interval.
- Use epinephrine-containing L.A with caution.
- If the patient is diabetic, ask the patient to test for diabetes and take prophylactic antibiotics.
- (Arrange juices and dextrose solution in case emergency hypoglycaemia occurs).
- Treat dry mouth with tart, candy or sugar free gum, sip of water or saliva substitute.
- Dry mouth increases the risk of dental caries, periodontal diseases and candidiasis.
- Advocate fluoride home treatment.
- Avoid use of alcohol containing mouth rinses. [10]

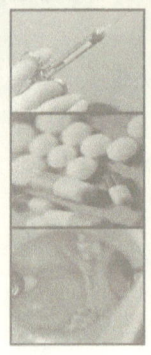

CHAPTER 12

ARBs (Angiotensin [II] receptor blockers)

CLASSIFICATION:

Irbesartan
Losartan
Olmesartan
Valsaratan
Telmisartan [2]

MODE OF ACTION:

They block angiotensin receptors so the mechanism is same as that of ACE-inhibitors. If they do not increase the level of bradykinin, side effect of dry cough is reduced and they are attractive therapy for hypertensive diabetics. Moreover, the risk of angioedema is also reduced. [10]

INDIVIDUAL DRUGS:

LOSARTAN:

It is the prototype ARB.

Side effect:
Oral: dental pain, dry mouth

Dosages:
For hypertension: 50mg of dose daily.
Alternatively, 25 mg of daily dose is given to patient with diuretics.

Beta-adrenergic blocking agents:

See chapter 7 Beta Adrenergic blocking agents.

Alpha-adrenergic blocking agents:

See chapter 6 Alpha Adrenergic Blocking agents.

Calcium channel blockers:

See chapter 9 Calcium channel blockers.

Renin inhibitor:

Aliskiren is the only drug that inhibits renin. It is as effective as ACE-inhibitors, ARBs, and Thiazide diuretics.
It can be used along with other antihypertensive drugs.

Side effects:
Angioedema, diarrhoea and cough are most common side effects. However, it can cause hyperkalemia when used along with valsartan. [2]

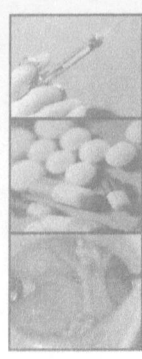

CHAPTER 13
Diuretics

Diuretics are those drugs, which increase the volume of urine produced by promoting the excretion of salts and water from kidney.

They are classified in to the following groups:

CLASSIFICATION:

Thiazide diuretics:
  Chlorothiazide
  Hydrochlorothiazide
  Polythiazide
  Bromothiazide

Loop diuretics
  Furosemide
  Bumetanide
  Torsemide
  Ethacrynic acid

Potassium sparing diuretics
    Amiloride
    Eplerenone
    Spironolactone
    Triamterene

Cabonic anhydrase inhibitor
    Acetazolamide

Osmotic diuretics
    Mannitol
    Urea [2]

Here, we will discuss only Thiazide diuretics and Loop diuretics.

THIAZIDE DIURETICS:

MODE OF ACTION:

Thiazide diuretics act on distal convulated tubule of kidney, thereby decrease Na^+ and Cl^- reabsorbtion resulting in retention of water in the tubule. Hence, cause diuresis.

INDICATIONS:

- Hypertension, it is useful for decreasing systolic and diastolic hypertension.
- Heart failure, as it causes depletion of fluid from body so Use for the treatment of heart failure.
  If Thiazide fails then loop diuretics may be useful.
- Renal stone, they prevent excretion of calcium ions in urine so useful for stone in urinary track.
- Oedema, they are also useful for oedema due to nephritis, nephrosis, heart failure, hepatic cirrhosis and due to corticosteroid and estrogen therapy.

SIDE EFFECTS:

Hpokalemia, lead to cardiac dysarrhythmia
Hyponatremia, lead to weakness and lethargy
Hypotension
Hyperglycemia
Hyperuricemia. (Which cause an increase uric acid in blood) [2]

Drug-Drug interaction:

Anaesthetics: thiazide may increase effect of anaesthetics.

Indomatacin: by inhibiting prostaglandin decreases effects of Thiazide.

Corticosteroids: enhances potassium loss because of potassium losing property of both.

Muscle relaxant-non depolarizing: increases effect of muscle relaxant due to hypokalemia effect.

INDIVIDUAL DRUGS:

Hydrochlorothiazide:

Additional side effects:

1. Toxic epidermal necrolysis
2. Stevens-Johnson syndrome erythema multiforme anaphylactic reactions
3. Respiratory distress includes pneumonitis and pulmonary oedema.

Dosage:

As a Diuretic, 25-200 mg/day initially for several days then increase upto 25-100 mg/day.

As Anti-hypertensive, 25 mg/day initial dose Then it may increase to 50 mg/day in daily divided doses.

DENTAL CONSIDERATION:

- Before commencement, any dental procedure Asses vital signs because of having cardiovascular side effects.
- For the heart patients Schedule early morning appointment in order to reduce anxiety.
- Use anxiety reduction protocol for anxious patient particularly with hypertension or HF.
- Consult patient's primary care physician before starting any dental procedure.
- Advise prothrombin and thrombin time for patients on anticoagulant therapy.
- Patient who is taking thiazide diuretics Measure his/her K^+ level of blood.
- Ask patient to avoid taking caffeine-containing beverages. [10]

LOOP DIURETICS:

MODE OF ACTION:

Loop diuretics inhibit the co-transport of $Na^+/K^+/2\ Cl^-$ at the ascending loop of Henle thus leading to retention of salt and water in the lumen. They are the most efficacious of diuretics. [2]

INDICATION:

Use for acute pulmonary oedema mostly due to HF.
Also use for hyperkalemia and hypercalcemia.

SIDE EFFECTS:

- Excessive dehydration may cause cardiovascular collapse, vascular thrombosis and embolism.
- Ototoxicity including tinnitius, vertigo and hearing loss is particular with ethacrynic acid when used along with some antibiotics especially aminoglycosides.
- Hypokalemia, loss of potassium ion from cells for exchange of hydrogen ion results in hypokalemic alkalosis. This can be warded-off by use of potassium sparing diuretics or use of potassium ion supplement.
- Hyperuricaemia, increase in uric acid in blood can occur by use of furosemide and ethacrynic acid that compete with uric acid for renal tubules thus blocking uric acid secretion leading to accumulation of uric acid in body ultimately leading to gouty attack.
- Hypomagnesemia, decrease in magnesium ion can occur when loop diuretic is used without supplement of magnesium intake from diet.(e-g: green leafy vegetables, bananas, peas etc)

INDIVIDUAL DRUGS:

Furosemide:

Indications:

- Use for oedema caused by CHF.
- Use for ascites.
- Use for acute pulmonary oedema, in IV form.
- Use for nephritic syndrome.
- Use for hepatic cirrhosis.
- Also use for hypertension in conjunction with spironolactone, triamterene and other diuretics.

Dosages:

Availability: 20, 40 and 80 mg tablets.

For oedema:

Dose 20-40 mg per day. The dose should not increase from 600 mg daily.

For hypertension:

Initially 40 mg b.i.d, then adjust according to response.

For CHF or chronic renal failure:

Dose is 2-2.5 g daily.

For acute pulmonary oedema:

Initially 40 mg is given over 1-2 minutes. Then if response is inadequate after 1 hour give 80 mg over 1-2 minutes. [10]

DENTAL CONSIDERATION:

For hypertensive patients (In general)

- Monitor vital signs particularly blood pressure of a patient.
- If patient with antihypertensive therapy has controlled blood pressure then start dental procedure.
- When patient has systolic blood pressure > 140 mm of Hg and diastolic > 90 mm of Hg, go for dental procedure but with the following precautions.

  1. Use anxiety reduction protocol.
  2. Donot exceed epinephrine dose of more than 0.04 mg with local anaesthetics.
  3. Avoid rapid posture changes of patient who takes drugs that cause vasodilation.
  4. Give local anaesthesia in supine position.
  5. Avoid administration of sodium containing solutions. [8]

- If patient has systolic blood pressure greater than 200 mm of Hg and diastolic greater than 110 mm of Hg.

Then,

1. Defer elective dental treatment until hypertension is better controlled.
2. Consider referral to a specialist for an emergency problem. [8]

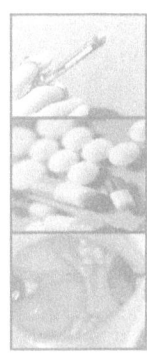

CHAPTER 14

Nitrates/ Nitrites

They are a class of drugs used as *coronary vasodilator* (for the treatment and prevention of angina).

CLASSIFICATION:

Organic nitrates:
Isosorbide dinitrate
Isosorbide mononitrate
Nitroglycerin (Glyceryl trinitrate)

MODE AND MECHANISM OF ACTION:

These drugs respond to angina pectoris in two ways; 1) by relaxation of coronary arteries, which increases blood flow to the myocardium, and 2) by relaxation of veins, which causes pooling of blood in venous system that in turns decreases the preload (venous return to the heart) ultimately reducing myocardial oxygen demand.

Nitroglycerin is thought to relax vascular smooth muscles by intracellular conversion into nitrite ions, then into nitric oxide that in turn converts into guanylate cyclase and increases the cell cyclic (GMP) guanosine monophosphate. Elevated cGMP leads to dephosphorylation of the myosin light chain, resulting in vascular smooth muscle relaxation.

Onset of action:

Nitroglycerin = 2 minutes (via sublingual)
= 35 minutes (via oral)
Isosorbide dinitrate = 5 minutes (via sublingual)
= 30 minutes (via oral)
Isosorbide mononitrate = 30 minutes (via oral)

Duration of action:

Nitroglycerin = 25 minutes (via sublingual)
= 4-8 hrs (via oral)
Isosorbide dinitrate = 1 hour (via sublingual)
= 8 hrs (via oral)
Isosorbide mononitrate =12 hours (via oral)

INDICATIONS:

- Use for patients with acute angina attack. (sublingually)
- Use as a prophylaxis of chronic angina pectoris.
- Use IV to decrease blood pressure during surgical procedure, which causes hypertension.
- Use as an adjunctive therapy for hypertensive patient and with CHF associated with MI.

SIDE EFFECTS:

- Most common side effect is headache.

- High doses may cause postural hypotension, hot flushing and tachycardia.
- Topical use may cause peripheral oedema and contact dermatitis.
- It also causes haemolytic anaemia.
- Oral: dry mouth, burning sensation

INDIVIDUAL DRUG:

Glyceryl trinitrate: (Nitroglycerin)

Dosages:
For termination of acute attack, 1 or 2 metered dose (400-800 mg) on or under the tongue repeat after every 5 minutes until acute attack subsides.

As a prophylaxis for acute attack, 1 or 2 metered doses 10-15 minutes before starting an activity that may precipitate acute Anginal attack.

DENTAL CONSIDERATION:

- Before commencement of any dental procedure, Asses vital signs of patient
- Evaluate anxious level of the patient; if severe, we can start with anti anxiety drugs like diazepam, clonazepam or nitrous oxide 1 hour before starting dental treatment.
- While giving local anaesthesia, be cautious about the content of L.A (Epinephrine) either give plan L.A or give with minimal dose of epinephrine that's not exceed from 0.04 mg per appointment.
- Give L.A injection in supine position in order to avoid syncope.
- Upright the patient slowly after giving L.A with an interval of 2 minutes in between in order to avoid postural hypotension.

- Make sure that Nitroglycerin drug is easily accessible in case angina attacks precipitate during dental procedure.
- Also check if the patient is on anticoagulant therapy or not, in which case consult primary care physician before starting any invasive procedure, e-g extraction.
- Manage dry mouth with tart, sugar free gum and/or saliva substitute.
- Avoid prescribing alcohol containing mouth rinses.
- Also, avoid taking caffeine-containing beverages. [10]

DRUGS EFFECTING BLOOD

These drugs fall into three categories 1) those drugs, which inhibit thrombo-embolism 2) those drugs that stop bleeding and 3) those drugs that treat anaemia.

Drugs that treat thrombo-embolism are mostly encountered while those stop bleeding are also important from dental point of view.

Thrombus is an unwanted clot of blood that remains adhere to blood vessel wall whereas embolus is an unwanted clot of blood that floats in the vessels. Both are dangerous as they may occlude blood flow to an organ resulting in ischemia and ultimately death of the tissue. Diseases caused by this phenomenon include **MI, Deep vein thrombosis, cerebral ischemia (stroke) and pulmonary embolism.**

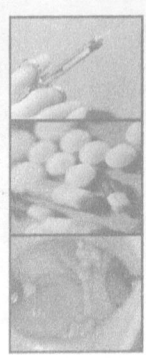

CHAPTER 15

Platelet Aggregation Inhibitors

This class of drug fall into the first category "drugs that affect thrombo-embolism".

CLASSIFICATION:

Aspirin
Clopidogrel
Ticlopidine
Abciximab

Normal mechanism of blood clotting:

1. Prostacyclin (prostaglandin I_2) and nitric oxide is released from intact endothelium, which stops activation of resting platelets.
2. Prostacyclin bind to resting platelets cause an increase in intracellular cAMP and decrease in Calcium ion release from the platelets.
3. So platelets are not activated.

4. When there is damage to the blood vessel either by cut or incision or by any mean, subendothelial collagen is exposed in the wall of blood vessels.

5. This collagen also release chemical mediators like ADP, thromboaxane A2, serotonin, platelet-activating factor (PAF) and thrombin.

6. These mediators bind to resting platelets and cause them to activate.

7. There is decrease in cAMP and increase in calcium ion release, which ultimately release further granules from the activated platelets.

8. Calcium ions do the following actions, 1. Release of platelet granules; 2. Activation of thromboaxane A2 synthesis; 3. Activation of glycoprotein receptor (GPIlb/IIIa receptors). Fibrinogen binds with GPIlb/IIIa receptor on two different platelets thus does cross-linking of platelets.

9. Injured tissues lead to local cascade of coagulation by tissue factor cause formation of clotting factor (IIa), thrombin. Thrombin catalyzes hydrolysis of fibrinogen into fibrin.

10. This results in formation of platelet-fibrin plug.

11. During plug formation, plasminogen is locally converted into plasmin (this is locally done by plasminogen activator) which limits the clotting mechanism. Therefore limiting the growth of clot and dissolves the fibrin network as the wound heals. [2]

MECHANISM OF ACTION:

Aspirin inhibits thromboaxane A_2 from arachidonic acid (which is produced from membrane phospholipid by platelet membrane phospholipase) by irreversible acetylation of serine group, which block the arachidonate to the active site thus inhibiting COX-1, which ultimately inhibits platelet aggregation. The inhibition effect of aspirin on thromboaxane A_2 lasts until the life of anucleate platelets that is 7-10 days.

Clopidogrel and *Ticlopidine,* they inhibit binding of ADP to its respective receptor on platelet membrane thus inhibiting activation of GPIIb/IIIa receptor, ultimately no fibrinogen binds to GPIIb/IIIa receptor and no cross linking of platelets occur.

INDICATIONS:

- Use as a prophylaxis for thromboembolic diseases like coronary syndrome (unstable angina, non-Q-wave MI).
- Use for patients with recent attack of MI, Stroke or established peripheral arterial diseases.
- Clopidogrel is a preferred drug for ischemic heart diseases.

SIDE EFFECTS:

- They prolong the bleeding time.
- Neutropenia/ Agranulocytosis
- Thrombotic thrombocytopenic purpura (TTP)
- Aplastic anaemia

Drug-Drug interaction:

Ibuprofen; when use concomitantly with aspirin, ibuprofen competes for the active site of serine thus block platelet inhibiting action of aspirin.

If at all use with aspirin, Aspirin should be taken either 30 minutes before taking ibuprofen or wait for 8 hours after the use of ibuprofen then take aspirin. [10]

INDIVIDUAL DRUGS:

1. **Aspirin:**
   Tablets: 75mg, 81 mg, 165 mg, 325 mg, 500 mg (enteric coated)
   Capsules: 325, 500 mg

Dosage:

loading dose 325 mg; maintenance dose 75mg per day.
Or ingestion of 325 mg every other day has also been shown
to reduce the risk of MI.

2. Ticlopidine

It is good for patients who cannot tolerate aspirin.

Adverse effects:

Nausea, dyspepsia and diarrhoea

Haemorrhage.

Leucopoenia

Dosage:

250 mg dose b.i.d [10]

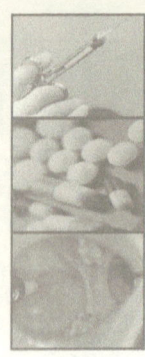

CHAPTER 16

Anticoagulants

They are the class of drugs use to prevent clotting of blood. They also come under the heading of first category "Drugs which inhibit thrombo-embolism".

CLASSIFICATION:

Heparin
Warfarin
Dalteparin
Enoxaparin
Argatroban

Normal blood Coagulation:

1. When blood vessel is injured and platelet plug is formed as mentioned in chapter 15. Fibrinogen needs thrombin formation in order to convert into fibrin.
2. For thrombin formation, there are two pathways extrinsic and intrinsic pathways.

3. In extrinsic pathway the triggering factors are damaged (activated) endothelium, subendothelial fibroblast, subendothelial smooth muscle cells and activated leukocytes.

4. In extrinsic pathway factor, VII is activated by tissue factor and thromboplastin (as produced by triggering factors in point 3.)

5. In intrinsic pathway, the triggering factors are glass and/or highly charged surfaces.

6. In intrinsic pathway factor, XII is activated when it meets charged surface containing phospholipid.

7. Because of both pathways, ultimately factor X is activated and X_a is formed.

8. This X_a converts prothrombin (II) into thrombin (II_a). This activated thrombin converts fibrinogen into fibrin.

9. A number of factors are responsible to keep this coagulation restricted to the site of vessel injury; they include protein S, protein C, anti-thrombin III and tissue factor pathway inhibitor.

   (Anti coagulant drugs act to activate these factors to inhibit Coagulation). [2]

MODE OF ACTION:

Heparin is also known as thrombin inhibitor; binds with anti-thrombin III accelerate its action to bind with *thrombin and factor Xa* thus inhibiting the action of coagulation factors. LMWHs are also available, which is a fragment of unfractionated Heparin, also binds with anti-thrombin III thus acting as a catalyst to bind fast with Factor Xa but not with thrombin.

Warfarin the coumarin anticoagulant, acts by antagonizing the effect of co-factor vitamin K. Vitamin K is essential for *the* synthesis of the following clotting factors (Factor II, Factor VI, Factor IX and Factor

X) in the liver. Therefore, Warfarin interferes with the synthesis of clotting factors.

INDICATIONS:

Heparin: (have rapid onset of action)

- Use for acute deep vein thrombosis.
- Use for Pulmonary embolism
- Use as a prophylaxis for postoperative venous thrombosis and for acute phase of MI.
- Also Use in pregnant patients with prosthetic heart valves or venous thromboembolism because heparin and LMWHs donot cross the placenta.
- LMWHs are subsequently followed by heparin (because heparin are rapidly terminated on suspension of therapy) they are mostly injected subcutaneously.

Warfarin:

- Use as a prophylaxis for MI, Prosthetic heart valves and chronic atrial fibrillation.

Use for acute deep vein thrombosis and pulmonary embolism after initial therapy of Heparin.

ADVERSE EFFECTS:

See section on Individual Drugs below.

INDIVIDUAL DRUGS:

1. **Heparin:**
   Adverse effects:

Bleeding disorder;
Oral: bleeding from gums
Bleeding from nose
Bleeding from intestine
Allergic reaction;
Urticaria
Fever
Chills
Anaphylaxis
Thrombocytopenia;
Decrease in platelet count is also observed in patient with heparin therapy.
Osteoporosis;
It is observed in-patient with long-term heparin therapy.

Dosages:
IV infusion; initial bolus injection 5000-10,000 units followed by 900 units /hour.

2. **Warfarin:**
   Adverse effects:
   Bleeding disorder;
   Patients taking Warfarin have frequent bleeding problem such as
   Oral: bleeding from gums
   Bleeding from nose
   Bleeding from intestine

Dosages:
Action of Warfarin is delayed.
Initial dose of 5-10 mg daily is maintained for week in order to Increase prothrombin time by 25% of normal value.

DENTAL CONSIDERATION:

- Take complete history of drugs before commencement of any dental procedure.
- If patient is taking any of the anticoagulants consult primary care physician to stop the drug for at least 3-5 days.
- Monitor partial thromboplastin time PTT; (as in case of heparin it increases 2-2.5 times that of control value) and prothrombin time PT (which in case of Warfarin is increased by 25%).
- Notify the dentist if bleeding from gums, sores or any oral lesion occurs.
- Refer patient to the periodontologist for gum bleeding problems.
- Avoid taking drugs that have anticoagulant effects like salicylates, NSAIDS and steroids.
- Prescribe soft bristle toothbrush to patient, if bleeding problem persists.
- Ensure the use of good oral hygiene in order to prevent further gingival inflammation and soft tissue injury. [10]

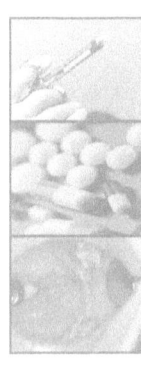

CHAPTER 17

Drugs for treatment of bleeding

They are divided into four groups

CLASSIFICATION:

Blood and its derivatives:

    Cryoprecipitate

    Novasevan

    FEIBA (factor VIII inhibitor by passing activity)

    Desmopressin Acetate

    Autoplex

    Factor VIII

    Factor IX

    Factor X

Vitamin K preparations:

    Natural Vitamin K1 (phytonadione)

    Natural Vitamin K2 (Menaquinone)

    Synthetic Vitamin K3 (Menadione)

<u>Fibrinolytic inhibitors:</u>
Aminocaproic acid
Tranexamic acid

<u>Heparin Antagonist:</u>
Protamine sulfate [3]

MODE OF ACTION:

- Aminocaproic acid and tranexamic acid inhibit plasminogen activation.
- Protamine sulfate antagonizes the action of anticoagulant Heparin.
- FFP contains all coagulation factors and is useful for patient with clotting factor deficiency.
- Cryoprecipitate contains Factor VII c, von willibrand factor (VWF) and fibrinogen, so useful in patients with DIC and other conditions where the fibrinogen level is very low.

INDICATIONS:

For bleeding disorder due to above-mentioned reasons and/ or excessive bleeding, that occurs during surgical procedure and is difficult to stop.

In dentistry, bleeding is common complication in post-extraction cases.

ADVERSE EFFECTS:

They may lead to thrombo-embolic events.

INDIVIDUAL DRUGS:

1. **Aminocaproic acid:**
   It is given PO 6 g q.i.d (or slowly intravenously)
   Its absorption is rapid and excretion is in the urine.
   It is a competitive inhibitor of plasminogen activator.
   It is use in bleeding disorders like:
   Haemophilia
   Fibrinolytic drugs induced bleeding &
   Use for prophylaxis of recurrent bleeding from intracranial aneurysm.

2. **Tranexamic acid:** (most commonly used in dentistry)
   It is an analogue of Aminocaproic acid.
   It is given PO.
   It inhibits fibrinolysis.
   It can be used to prevent bleeding or bleeding associated with excessive fibrinolysis for example, in dental extraction of a patient with Haemophilia or patient with menorrhagia.

3. **Protamine sulfate:**
   It acts as an antidote for heparin.

4. **Vitamin K**
   Vitamin K is a fat-soluble vitamin and confers the activity of prothrombin, Factor VII, Factor IV and Factor X.
   There are three types;
   Vitamin K_1 is found in food and is called phytonadione.
   Vitamin K_2 is found in human intestine secreted by intestinal bacteria and is called menaquinone.
   Vitamin K_3 is a synthetic vitamin K known as menadione.
   Response to vitamin K is slow and requiring 24 hours.

Indications:

- Patient on excess Warfarin (where there is depression of prothrombin activity). Vitamin K is an antidote for oral anticoagulant Warfarin.
- Use on patient with vitamin K deficiency.

Availability:

5 mg tablets, 50mg ampules. [3]

DENTAL CONSIDERATION:

- Take full history from patient before going for extraction or any other surgical procedure.
- If patient is taking anticoagulants then go for checking INR. This value takes into account the patient's prothrombin time and the standardized control.
- If the value is 2.5 or less, go for extraction.
- If the value is upto 3.0, then take high precaution while extracting.
- Stop the drug 5 days before extraction then resume them a day after an extraction in case the bleeding does not persist.
- If value of INR is above 3.0, then defer the extraction procedure and consult the patient's primary care physician.
- In case post extraction bleeding does not stop after 24 hours, then place absorbable gelatine sponge (Gelfoam) in the socket and suture it.
- Another material that can be used instead of Gelfoam is surgicel (oxidized regenerated cellulose) it promotes coagulation better than absorbable gelatin sponge. [8]
- If bleeding is severe dentist can apply liquid preparation of thrombin onto gelatin sponge, this thrombin bypasses all the

steps in coagulation cascade and helps to convert fibrinogen into fibrin quickly.

- Collagen; (microfibular collagen) is also the material of choice because it promotes platelet aggregation and thereby accelerates coagulation.
- Regular follow up is mandatory in order to monitor bleeding problem. [8]

ANALGESICS

Analgesics are those drugs that are use to relief pain. Mild to Moderate pain gets relive by NSAIDS (e-g Aspirin, ibuprofen) and Acetaminophen while moderate to severe pain is relieved by Opioids (e-g Morphine, Codeine).

Chapter 18 is about NSAIDS, Chapter 19 discusses Acetaminophen while Chapter 20 is about Opioids.

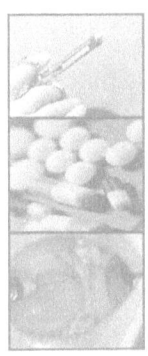

CHAPTER 18

NSAIDS

They are Non-steroidal anti-inflammatory drugs. They are also known as non-narcotic analgesics.

CLASSIFICATION:

COX-1 & COX-2 Inhibitors
   Diclofenac
   Etodolac
   Fenoprofen
   Flurbiprofen
   Ibuprofen
   Indomatacin
   Ketoprofen
   Ketorolac
   Meclofenamate
   Mefenamic acid
   Naproxen
   Oxaprozin
   Piroxicam
   Sulindac
   Aspirin [2]

COX-2 Inhibitor
Celecoxib

MECHANISM OF ACTION:

NSAID drugs inhibit the production of prostaglandin via blocking cyclooxygenase pathway.

Cyclooxygenase pathway:

In this pathway, two enzymes are responsible COX-1 (cyclooxygenase 1) and COX-2 (cyclooxygenase 2).

COX-1 is responsible for physiologic production of prostaglandin such as prostaglandin used for gastric protection, kidney function, vascular homeostasis and platelet aggregation While COX-2 is responsible for production of PG in inflamed tissue of the body.

From tissues cell membrane, which contains phospholipids, arachidonic acid forms by an enzyme phospholipase. This arachidonic acid then converts into PG G_2 via cyclooxygenase pathway.

Prostaglandin G_2 is then converted into prostaglandin H_2 which ultimately Gets convert into prostacyclin (prostaglandin I2), thromboaxane A2 (TX A2) and PG D2 and PG E2.

INDICATIONS:

NSAIDs have three major therapeutic effects.

1. Anti-inflammatory:
   They inhibit cyclooxygenase pathway thus decrease production of prostaglandin at the site of inflammation.

2. Analgesic:
   Prostaglandin E2 is thought to sensitize the nerve endings to mediators like bradykinin, histamine etc as they are produced during inflammation. Therefore, NSAIDs decrease the nerve sensitivity in this way and reduce pain.

3. Anti-pyretic:
   When pyrogens from white cells are activated as a result of infection they stimulate PGE2 which increases the set point of anterior hypothalamic regulatory centre in the brain causing fever. So NSAIDs inhibit these prostaglandin syntheses.
   Other indications include:

   - Topically, salicylic acid is use for corns, calluses and warts.
   - Aspirin is use in low doses as a prophylaxis against sudden death cause by acute MI, transient ischemic attacks and stroke.
   - Aspirin is also use for patients with chronic stable angina as a prophylaxis for MI. [3]

ADVERSE EFFECTS:

Oral: dry mouth, salivation, stomatitis, gingival ulcers and glossitis
GI: peptic ulceration and/or duodenal ulcer
Respiratory: aggravate asthma and hay fever
Kidney: chronic tubulointerstitial nephritis
Blood: prolongs the bleeding time.
Allergy: including urticaria, bronchospasm and angioedema

Contraindications:

Pregnancy; as it causes unnecessarily prolongation of labor by blocking prostaglandin synthesis therefore contraindicated in third trimester. It also cause premature ductus arteriosus in newborn so, contraindicated in first trimester. It also prevents implantation of fertilized egg (therefore it should not be given to new couple desiring to conceive a child).
Breast-feeding; as salicylates are secreted in milk therefore, they should be avoided during breast-feeding.

Asthma; NSAIDs block the cyclooxygenase pathway so the alternate pathway becomes predominated that is, Lipooxygenase pathway in which leukotriene is produced (chemical mediators responsible for asthma).

Peptic ulceration; patients who have gastric ulceration problem should avoid using NSAIDs if at all necessary it should be used in combination with prostaglandin analogue (misoprostol). Arthrotec is commercially used drug, which contains diclofenac & misoprostol.

Nephrotic syndrome; patient with kidney problem such as proteinuria and hypoalbuminemea should avoid using NSAIDs at all because they are highly nephrotoxic.

INDIVIDUAL DRUGS:

1. **Celecoxib:**
   Availability: 100-200 mg tablets
   Dosage: 200 mg dose PO b.i.d

2. **Diclofenac:**
   Availability: 50mg tablets
   Dosage: 50mg PO t.i.d

3. **Ibuprofen:**
   Availability: 200, 400 & 600 mg tablets.
   Dosage: 400 mg dose PO every 4-6 hours.

4. **Indomatacin:**
   Availability: 25 and 50 mg capsules
   Dosage: 25-50 mg dose PO t.i.d

5. **Piroxicam:**
   Availability: 10-20 mg capsules
   Dosage: 20 mg dose PO q.i.d

6. **Aspirin:**
   Availability: 75, 325 & 500 mg tablets
   Dosage: 300-600 mg dose (as anti-inflammatory) [3]

DENTAL CONSIDERATION:

- Dry mouth may predispose patient to dental caries, periodontal disease and candidiasis.
- Ask the patient to avoid aspirin containing drugs as it may cause ulceration on oral mucosa.
- Avoid using OTC drugs by patient.
- Take care, while prescribing NSAID drugs to patient with gastric ulceration.
- NSAIDs are widely used analgesics for dental pain (like reversible or irreversible pulpitus).
- Patient should take NSAIDs with full glass of water or milk or with prescribed antacids, and then patient should remain upright for 30 minutes in order to avoid gastric irritation and chest burning.
- Dentist can prescribe arthrotec (diclofenac plus misoprostol) combination, for it will protect the stomach from gastric acid.
- If NSAID is contraindicated then dentist should prescribe alternative that is Acetaminophen.
- Acetaminophen plus codeine is also another alternative for dental pain. [11]

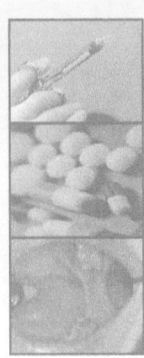

CHAPTER 19
Acetaminophen

It is a weak prostaglandin inhibitor and has weak or no anti-inflammatory effect.

MODE OF ACTION:

It inhibits synthesis of prostaglandin in CNS but it has little effect on peripheral PG, which is responsible for inflammation. It also has an effect on hypothalamus heat regulating centre to increase sweating and cause vasodilation.

INDICATIONS:

- It is a potent anti-pyretic and analgesic.
- It is useful in all conditions where we use aspirin for controlling pain and fever.
- It is also use to control dental pain but when dental pain is associated with inflammation like cellulitus Acetaminophen plays no role as an anti-inflammatory.

- It is also a drug of choice in children with viral infections and fever, for it does not cause Reye's syndrome as opposed to aspirin.

ADVERSE EFFECTS:

Liver: hepatic necrosis, a life threatening condition can result from high doses. FHF (jaundice appears within 2 weeks of previously normal liver) can occur followed by encephalopathy and GI bleeding.

CNS: On CNS, it causes dizziness and drowsiness.

Allergy: skin rashes and minor allergic reactions can occur rarely.

Kidney: Renal tubular necrosis may be a consequence of prolong use of large doses.

Metabolic: hypoglycaemic coma may occur rarely with prolong use of large doses.

INDIVIDUAL DRUGS:

Acetaminophen:

Availability: 500 mg tablet.

Dosage: 500 mg-1g dose q.i.d.

Other combination is with Codeine [8]

In this combination Acetaminophen, 500 mg & codeine 15 mg are present (available in Pakistan by name of Codogesic).

Acetaminophen along with codeine has a potent analgesic effect and used commonly for severe sharp lacerating pain of tooth (irreversible pulpitus).

DENTAL CONSIDERATION:

- Asses need for use of acetaminophen.
- We should evaluate patient using acetaminophen on long-term therapy, for blood dyscrasias.

- Acetaminophen is prescribed for children with dental pain.
- If patient has complaint of burning chest or tightness of chest then do prescribe acetaminophen instead of NSAIDs.
- If patient is suffering with emergency dental pain *(Signs of emergency dental pain are, "they affect the patient normal daily life activities, pain does not subside by NSAIDs and pain history is less than two days")* then do prescribe acetaminophen plus codeine.[11]

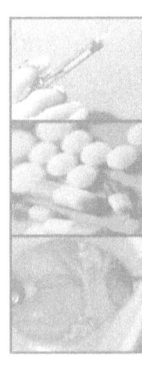

CHAPTER 20

Opioids

Opioids are the class of drugs derived from opium. The naturally occurring opioid is known as opiate.

Morphine is the naturally occurring drug. Opiate drugs depress CNS, relieve pain, suppress coughing and stimulate vomiting.

CLASSIFICATION:

Strong agonist:
Morphine
Oxycodone
Fentanyl
Alfentanil
Sufentanil
Methadone
Mepiridine

Low agonist:
Codeine
Propoxyphene [3]

MECHANISM OF ACTION:

Opioid agonists bind to receptors (mu, delta and kappa) located in the brain and spinal cord that are responsible for transmission and modulation of pain.

These receptors belong to a family known as 'G-protein coupled receptors' *see chapter 3 Interaction of Drugs with Receptors*.

Morphine is a typical of all drugs and binds to mu receptor. This is primarily responsible for analgesia, euphoria, respiratory depression and physiological dependence of morphine.

Cellular action:

Opioids act either on presynaptic neurons, when they bind to its receptor they close calcium ion channel, which ultimately reduces the release of neurotransmitters (serotonin, glutamate, acetylcholine, nor-epinephrine and substance P). On the other hand, they act on receptors on post synaptic neurons, hyperpolarize them by opening potassium channel. Thus ultimately reducing or nullifying pain transmission.

Distribution of Receptors:

They generally occur in five different areas of CNS.

1. Brian stem (influence cough, respiration, blood pressure and control of stomach secretion). medial thalamus (influence pain which is emotionally affected)
2. Spinal cord (present in substantia gelatinosa location here they weaken the afferent painful stimuli).
3. Hypothalamus (influences neuroendocrine secretion).
4. Limbic system (present in amygdala location here influence more of emotional behaviour rather than analgesic action). [3]

In addition, these opiate receptors are also present on peripheral neurons where they also contribute to analgesic effect by inhibiting release of neurotransmitter by blocking the calcium ions channels.

Opioid receptors are of the following types:

1. Mu μ: stimulation of mu receptors produces mainly analgesia, sedation, euphoria, respiratory depression and constipation.
2. Kappa κ: stimulation of kappa receptor produces analgesia.
3. Delta: their stimulation produces analgesia, respiratory depression and reduced gastrointestinal motility. [3]

INDICATIONS:

- They are useful for controlling severe constant pain and in particular, when sleep induction is necessary.
- They are use along with Acetaminophen, particularly the codeine to synergise the effect of analgesia. For example, sharp irreversible pulpitus pain.
- They are also efficacious in subside the pain of cancer.
- They are also use to relieve renal and biliary colic pain.
- They are also useful for suppression of cough; however, more useful drugs are available that have antitussive property such as dextromethorphan, which has no more analgesic or addictive effect.
- Because of their sedative, anxyolitic and analgesic properties, they are use as pre-operative analgesic particularly in cardiovascular surgery.
- IV administration of morphine in relieving dyspnea due to acute pulmonary oedema is remarkable exact mechanism is unknown. However, it is assume that dyspnea gets relive by its vasodilating activity (i-e reducing the pre-load and after-load).

SIDE EFFECTS:

- Sever respiratory depression due its effect on respiratory centre in brain stem.
- Potential for addiction (withdrawal symptoms may occur 6-10 hours after the last dose of morphine or heroin).
- Signs and symptoms of withdrawal *(abstinence syndrome)* are lacrimation, yawning, chills, gooseflesh (piloerection), hyperventilation, hyperthermia anxiety, vomiting, diarrhoea, and hostility.
- Sedation
- Constipation
- Urinary retention is particularly with BPH.
- Therapeutic dose may cause flushing and warming of skin followed by sweating and itching.
- In the oral cavity, it can cause dry mouth. [10]

Contraindications:

1. Asthma, emphysema, diabetic ketoacidosis epilepsy
2. Addison's disease hepatic cirrhosis

INDIVIDUAL DRUGS:

1. **Codeine: (sulfate / phosphate)**
    Availability: 15, 30 and 60 mg tablets.
    Parenteral: 30-60 mg/ml for IM, IV & SC. [3]
    Dosage: for analgesia, 15-60 mg dose t.i.d or q.i.d
    For cough, 10-20 mg dose q.i.d

2. **Morphine (sulfate)**
    Availability: 10, 15 & 30 mg tablets. [3]
    Parenteral 10, 20, & 100 mg /5 ml
    Dosage: 10 mg dose (Approx.)

3. **Fentanyl**
   Availability: 50 µgram /ml for injection.
   Dosage:
   Pre-operatively give 0.05-0.1 mg dose IM 30-60 minutes before the start of surgery.
   As adjunct to regional anaesthesia, give 0.05-0.1 mg IM or IV over 1-2 minutes when indicated.
   Post-operatively give 0.05-0.1 mg dose repeatedly 1-2 hours for control of pain.

4. **Oxycodone**
   Availability: 5 mg tablet.
   Parenteral: 1-20 mg/ml solution
   Combination:

   - Oxycodone/Acetaminophen
     This combination includes 5 mg Oxycodone plus 500 mg acetaminophen.
   Dosage:
     For dental pail (irreversible pulpitus) two tablets are given, so maximum dose of acetaminophen (i-e 1000 mg) achieved with 10 mg of oxycodone.
   - Oxycodone/Aspirin
     This combination includes 4.9 mg Oxycodone plus 325 mg aspirin. [3]

OPIOID ANTAGONISTS:

CLASSIFICATION:

Naloxone
Naltrexone

MODE OF ACTION:

Antagonists strongly bind to opiate receptors but donot activate them. Therefore, it strongly reverses the action of agonist binding as a result it induces opiates withdrawal symptoms. (In normal individual opioid antagonist produces no withdrawal symptoms).

INDICATIONS:

- To antagonize the effect of agonists like heroin and morphine
- They are use to reverse the effect of opioid overdose like coma and respiratory depression.

ADVERSE EFFECTS:

They induce withdrawal symptoms in opioid abusers.

INDIVIDUAL DRUGS:

1. **Naloxone:**
   IV injection antagonizes the action of opioid agonists and quickly relieve patient of respiratory depression and coma (within 30 seconds).
   Half-life: is 60-100 minutes.
   Availability: it is parenteraly available as 0.4 &1 mg/ml.

2. **Naltrexone:**
   It has longer duration of action than naloxone (i-e upto 48 hours), it antagonizes the action of injected heroin.
   Availability: it is available in 50mg tablet. [3]

DENTAL CONSIDERATION:

- Identify the cause of opioid therapy.
- Take history of opioids side effects like hot flushing and sweating.
- While giving L.A, make the patient supine and deliver L.A injection then upright him slowly over interval of 2 minutes.
- Opioid can cause sedation so NSAIDs are use as a synergistic pain reliever.
- Dry mouth predisposes patient to dental caries, periodontitis and candidiasis risk.
- Advocate fluoride home treatment to the patient.
- Avoid use of alcohol containing mouth rinses.
- Avoid use of caffeine containing beverages.
- Advocate evaluation of dental caries and periodontitis after every 6-month interval. [10]

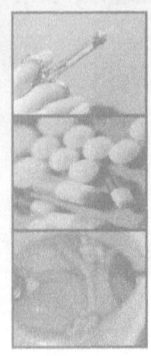

CHAPTER 21

Anti-Convulsants

They are the drugs use to prevent or reduce the severity and frequency of seizures in various types of epilepsy. They are also known as *anti-epileptic drugs*.

CLASSIFICATION:

Anti-convulsants:
    Phenytoin
    Mephenytoin
    Carbamazepine
    Oxcarbazepine
    Phenobarbital
    Lamotrigine
    Topiramate
    Felbamate
    Gabapentin
    Tiagabine

Benzodiazepines:
    Diazepam

Clonazepam
Clobazam

Epilepsy at a glance:

In epilepsy, there is sudden, excessive and synchronous electrical discharge from cerebral cortex of brain.

We classify epilepsy into two main types.

1) Partial
2) Generalized

1) Partial: This involves only a portion of brain such as one part of a lobe of one hemisphere.
   Signs and symptoms may include abnormal activity of a single limb or a group of muscle that is controlled by that particular brain area which is experiencing the disturbances.

2) Generalized: In this, abnormal electrical charges may produce in both hemisphere of brain. It is accompanied with loss of consciousness, tonic (continuous contraction) and clonic (rapid contraction and relaxation) phases along with depletion of glucose and energy stores.

MODE OF ACTION:

See section on Individual Drugs below.

INDICATIONS:

See section on Individual Drugs below.

ADVERSE EFFECTS:

See section on Individual Drugs below.

INDIVIDUAL DRUGS:

Phenytoin:

Mechanism of action:

It blocks the voltage-gated-Na^+ channels and hence slowing its rate of recovery in the brain. At higher dose, it also blocks voltage—gated-Ca^{++} ion channels hence interfere with the release of neurotransmitters.

Indications:

- In dentistry, it is mostly use for pain of nerve origin (i-e trigeminal neuralgia, glossopharyngeal neuralgia etc.)
- It is use for partial seizures.
- For generalized tonic-clonic seizures and for status epilepticus (a medical emergency in which there is continuous repeated seizures without recovery of consciousness between them).

Side effects:

Oral: In oral cavity, it produces *gingival hyperplasia*.

Chronic use may lead to vitamin D metabolism abnormality resulting in osteomalacia.

Nystagmus occurs due to loss of extra ocular pursuit movement.

Diplopia and ataxia are also common.

Rapid parenteral administration may cause severe CV effects including **hypotension, arrhythmias, cardiovascular collapse and heart block** as well as CNS depression.

Availability: 30, 100 mg capsules.
Parenterally it is given in a dose of 50mg /ml in IV injection. [3]

Dosages:

For trigeminal neuralgia, 100 mg t.i.d, then increase after 1 week to 100 mg q.i.d. maximum dose should not exceed 600 mg /day. [8]

New research has also shown that IV phenytoin has shown to subside with the pain for 10 months. The dose is 15 mg/kg, which is divided into two doses each one separated by 4 hours interval.

Carbamazepine:

Mode of action:

It blocks Na^+ channel in CNS, thus reducing the propagation of abnormal impulses in the brain from the focus of discharging electrical impulses.

Indications:

- For partial seizures
- Generalized tonic clonic seizures
- Typically use for Trigeminal neuralgia in dental office.

Side effects:

Oral: dry mouth, glossitis and stomatitis

Hematologic: idiosyncratic blood dyscrasias, including aplastic anaemia and granulocytosis (mostly seen in adults on therapy for trigeminal neuralgia and occurs after the first 4 months of the start of thereapy).

Idiosyncratic: *Erythematic skin rash* [10]

Others: hyponatremia, GI disturbance, unsteadiness, drowsiness, and water intoxication *Diplopia and Ataxia*

Availability:

It is available in 200 mg tablet and 100 mg chewable tablet.

Dosages:

Initial start with 200 mg t.i.d then may increase to q.i.d. maximum dose should not exceed more than 1200 mg /day.

New research has shown that concomitant use of baclofen increasing upto 60 mg, with subsequent reduction in carbamazepine dose is highly effective in relieving the pain.

DENTAL CONSIDERATION:

- Schedule an early appointment in the morning to reduce the stress and anxiety level in anxious patient.
- Patient on anticonvulsant drug therapy should have frequently gums evaluated for gingival hyperplasia.
- Patient at risk for gingival hyperplasia should be advice for keeping good oral hygiene, use of soft toothbrush, use of waxed dental floss daily and have regular check up from dentist.
- Patient with dry mouth is susceptible to dental caries, gingivitis and candidiasis infection.
- Use of fluoride home treatment should be advice to the patient.
- Patient on anticonvulsant drugs should have blood count check because of the possibility of idiosyncratic blood dyscrasias (symptoms include fever, sore throat, bleeding from gums and poor wound healing).

- If patient undergoes status epilepticus (medical emergency) during dental procedure, an immediate IV phenytoin injection should be made available and injected and the patient be send to hospital emergency quickly.
- If patient is diagnose with trigeminal neuralgia pain, then prescribe phenytoin or carbamazepine according to your assessment of patient.
- Avoid use of alcohol containing mouth rinses.
- Avoid use of caffeine containing beverages.
- Tart, sugar free chewing gums and/or saliva substitute is use to treat dry mouth. [10]

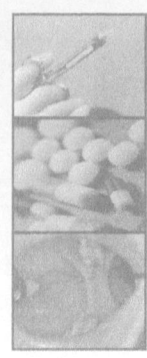

CHAPTER 22
Anxiolytics and Hypnotics

Anxiolytics are the class of drugs use to treat anxiety of various causes. They were formerly known as *minor tranquilizers*.

Hypnotics are the class of drugs that produces sleep by depressing brain function. They include benzodiazepines, anti-histamine (promethazine), zolpidem, zaleplon, zopiclone and Eszopiclone.

(Zaleplon and Zolpidem have neither anti-convulsant property nor muscle relaxation property).

Here we will discuss only Benzodiazepine in detail, which is relevant to dentistry.

CLASSIFICATION:

Benzodiazepines:
    Diazepam
    Lorazepam
    Alprazolam
    Clonazepam
    Chlordiazepoxide
    Quazepam
    Estazolam

Temazepam

Triazolam

MODE OF ACTION:

Benzodiazepines bind to GABA receptors in the CNS, making additive action to the conductance of Cl⁻ ion channels thus hyperpolarizing the neurons and make them difficult to depolarize. Hence, its inhibitory action is enhanced.

INDICATIONS:

1. For anxiety disorder: At low doses, they are useful for treating anxiety usually associated with depression and schizophrenia.
2. Muscular spasm: In dentistry, it is of particular importance, when muscles of mastication has undergone into spasm resulting in chronic pain and fatigue of TMJ. Benzodiazepine is in particular useful.
3. Seizures: Diazepam and lorazepam are use in treating status epilepticus. Whereas diazepam, chlordiazepoxide and oxazepam are use to treat alcohol withdrawal related seizure.
4. Sleep disorder: commonly use benzodiazepines are Flurazepam (long acting), Temazepam (intermediate acting) and Triazolam (short acting).

SIDE EFFECTS:

- Sedation: it can occur at very low doses even when they have no anti anxiety effect.
- Euphoria, impaired judgement, and loss of self-control can occur at doses use for anti-anxiety effect.
- Ataxia (unsteady gait and movement)

- Cognitive impairment (decreases long-term memory)
- Respiratory depression and sleep apnoea. [2]

Contraindications:

- Concomitant use of alcohol or any other CNS depressant drugs contraindicates use of benzodiazepines.
- Liver disease contraindicates its use.
- Acute-narrow angle glaucoma also contraindicates its use

INDIVIDUAL DRUGS:

1. **Diazepam:**
   Availability: 2, 5 and 10 mg tablets. [3]
   Parenterally, 5 mg/ml
   Dosages: 2-10 mg b.i.d—q.i.d, in debilitated patients 2-2.5 mg O.D or b.i.d
   For alcohol withdrawal, 10 mg t.i.d for 24 hours then reduce to 5 mg t.i.d
   For anxiety disorder 0.25-0.5 mg t.i.d

2. **Lorazepam:**
   Availability: 0.5, 1 and 2 mg tablets [3]
   Dosages: 1-3 mg b.i.d or t.i.d

3. **Alprazolam:**
   Availability: 0.25, 0.5 mg tablets. [3]
   Dosage: For anxiety disorder 0.25-0.5 mg t.i.d

DENTAL CONSIDERATION:

- Identify anxiety level and any contributing factor for anxiety.
- These drugs are use for conscious sedation in dentistry as a pharmacological anxiety reduction protocol.

- The protocol is to take oral medication by the patient 30-60 minutes before the start of oral procedure like extraction or any oral surgery.
- Diazepam (Valium) 2-10 mg or Lorazepam (Ativan) 1-4 mg or Alprazolam (Xanax) 0.25-0.5 mg can be given half to one hour before surgery.
- Have the patient escorted by attendant to dental office and to the dental chair.
- Schedule an early morning appointment to reduce waiting room time.
- Have a constant verbal communication with the patient to reduce his/her anxiety.
- Donot prescribe alcohol containing mouth rinses, for alcohol may aggravate the action of sedative-hypnotics.
- Donot stop taking the drug suddenly as it may cause rebound high level of anxiety and withdrawal symptoms like anorexia, vomiting, insomnia, muscle twitching, confusion and hallucination.

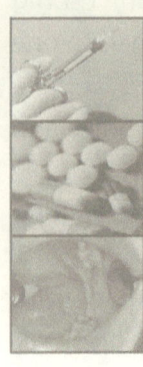

CHAPTER 23
Anti depressants

CLASSIFICATION

<u>Tricyclic antidepressant</u>
 Amitriptyline
 Nortriptyline
 Protriptyline
 Imipramine
 Desipramine
 Doxepin

<u>SSRIs</u>
 Citalopram
 Escitalopram
 Fluoxetine
 Paroxetine
 Sertratline [2]

MECHANISM OF ACTION:

Anti-depressant drugs enhance the effect of monoamines (serotonin and nor-epinephrine) in different sites of brain.

According to amine theory, depression is caused by deficiency of (nor-epinephrine or serotonin) monoamines in the brain. As opposed to mania which is caused by excess of these amines. However, this is still a theory because when antidepressant drug is administered it immediately affects the levels of amine but apparent affect on the patient is seen by 2-12 weeks of the administration of drug.

Tricyclic antidepressant drugs inhibit the re-uptake of serotonin plus nor-epinephrine by pre-synaptic neuron thus increasing the concentration of these amines in the synaptic cleft. This is useful for treating depression.

(Note: tricyclic antidepressants also act on other receptors like histaminic, muscarinic, serotonergic and alpha-adrenergic receptors).

(SSRIs selectively inhibit reuptake of serotonin by presynaptic neurons thus enhancing their concentration in the synaptic cleft). [3]

INDICATIONS:

- Use for endogenous and reactive *depression.*
- Use for *panic disorder* (condition featuring recurrent brief episodes of acute distress, mental confusion and fear of impending death). Benzodiazepines are the drugs of choice.
- Use for *Obsessive-compulsive disorder* (a recurrent thought, feeling or action that is unpleasant and provoke anxiety but cannot be got rid of. For example, repeatedly washing hands) mixed serotonin and nor-epinephrine uptake inhibitors are the drug of choice. [2]
- Use for *Chronic pain*, it has been widely used by clinician in pain clinics for chronic pain syndrome, fibromyalgia and chronic fatigue syndrome.

- Use in *dentistry*, it can be use to treat neuropathic pain and also pain of unknown origin, for example *trigeminal neuralgia* may or may not be associated with chronic headache or migraine.
- Use in *dentistry*, they are also used to treat chronic myofascial pain dysfunction syndrome (MFPDs). The doses are kept low such as Amitriptyline (10-25 mg at bedtime). This may improve sleep patterns, decrease bruxism, and result in decrease joint and muscle pain.

ADVERSE EFFECTS:

Sedation, sleepiness and additive effect with other sedative drugs

Antimuscarinic effect: blurred vision, constipation, urinary hesitancy and confusion

Adrenergic effect: tremor and insomnia

Cardiovascular effect: orthostatic hypotension and arrhythmias

Psychiatric effect: withdrawal syndrome and aggravation of psychosis

Metabolic effect: weight gain and sexual disturbances

Oral: dry mouth, stomatitis, glossitis, altered taste sensation and black tongue [10]

INDIVIDUAL DRUGS:

1). Amitriptyline:
Availability: 10, 25, 50, 75, 100 and 150 mg tablets.

Dosages:
As anti-depressant, 75-200 mg dose per day.
As analgesic for chronic trigeminal neuralgia, 10-300 mg dose per day.

2). Nortriptyline:

Availability: 10, 25, 50 and 75mg capsules.

Dosages:
As antidepressant 75-150 mg
As analgesic for trigeminal neuralgia, 10-150 mg dose per day.

3). Imipramine:

Availability: 10, 25, 50 mg tablets (hydrochloride)

Dosages:
As anti-depressant, 75-200 mg dose per day
As analgesic for trigeminal neuralgia 10-300 mg dose per day.

DENTAL CONSIDERATION:

- Monitor vital signs on every appointment because of cardiovascular side effects of tricyclic antidepressants.
- Use epinephrine-containing L.A with caution also, avoids use of epinephrine soaked gingival retraction cord.
- Dry mouth may predispose patient to dental caries, periodontal disease and candidiasis infection.
- Advocate fluoride home treatment.
- Avoid use of alcohol containing mouth rinses.
- Avoid use of caffeine containing beverages.
- Dentist can prescribe tricyclic anti-depressant to patients with chronic headaches and neuropathic pain after full evaluation and assessment.
- Donot use with diazepam as it may increase its sedative effects.
- Donot use with opioid analgesics as it may enhances the opioid induced respiratory depression.

- Donot use with anti-histamine as it may worsen dry mouth effect.
- *Avoid concomitant use with ethyl alcohol* as it may increase GI complication and decrease performance on motor skill tests; death has been reported. [10]

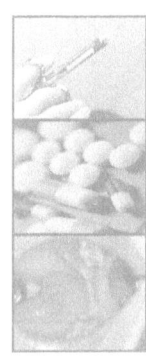

CHAPTER 24
Skeletal Muscle Relaxants

CLASSIFICATION:

CNS muscle relaxant:
    Diazepam
    Baclofen
    Carisoprodol
    Cyclobenzaprine
    Tizanidine
    See also chapter 22 Anxyolitic and Hypnotics

Neuromuscular blocking drugs:
    Non-depolarizing blockers:
    Tubocurarine
    Mivacurium
    Atracurium
    Pancuronium
    Vecuronium

    Depolarizing blockers:
    Succinyl choline

Neurotoxins:

Botulinum toxin

ß-bungarotoxin

MECHANISM OF ACTION:

Nicotine are the receptors on muscle cells, acetylcholine are the neurotransmitters at the neuromuscular junction.

Non-depolarizing drugs such as **tubocurarine** bind to nicotinic receptors thus blocking the binding of acetylcholine. At the same time they donot stimulate the receptor which lead to muscle relaxation by no depolarization occurrence at all. That is the sodium channel does not open.

Depolarizing blockers like **Succinyl choline** binds with nicotinic receptor blocks the action of acetylcholine, but do stimulate the receptor. The only difference between the Succinyl choline and acetylcholine is that acetylcholine gets degrade by acetyl-cholinesterase enzyme present at the synaptic cleft while Succinyl choline do not get degrade. So Succinyl choline initially cause small twitching of the muscles but later on, as it continue to bind with the receptor, continuous depolarization gives way to gradual repolarization as the sodium channel closes or get blocked.[1]

INDICATIONS:

- Use as an adjunctive drug with anaesthesia to induce muscle relaxation during surgery.
- Use when rapid endotracheal tube intubation is required during the induction of anaesthesia.
- Botulinum toxin is use to relieve muscle spasm (MFPDS) by intramuscular injection into the masseter muscle. [8] In addition, botulinum toxin is also use for the treatment of sialorrhoea, blepharospasm and urinary incontinence due to over activity of bladder.

- Use for acute muscle spasm of muscles of mastication (lateral pterygoid and medial pterygoid muscles).
- Use for acute myofascial pain dysfunction syndrome (TMJ disorder).

In the latter two indications diazepam, carisoprodol and cyclobenzaprine are the drugs of choice. [8]

SIDE EFFECTS:

Tubocurarine also releases histamine resulting in BP reduction, flushing and bronchoconstriction.

Hyperkalemia may occur in response to succinylcholine to such a level that cardiac arrest may occur.

Use of Succinyl choline may cause an increase in intraocular pressure.

Use of Succinyl choline may also cause an increase in intragastric pressure resulting in emesis, with the jeopardy of aspirating gastric content.

Following the use of Succinyl choline in surgery, patient may complain of muscle pain and in some patients muscle damage is been reported because of the presence of myoglobinurea.

Side effects of *botulinum toxin* include *dry mouth, blurred vision, dysphagia,* leading to progressive respiratory paralysis and parasympathetic and motor paralysis. [1]

INDIVIDUAL DRUGS:

1). Baclofen
Availability: 10, 20 mg tablets

Dosages:
For (MFPDS) 5-10 mg t.i.d may be increase gradually by 15 mg increments at 3 days interval until pain relief is achieved.

2). Carisoprodol
Availability: 350 mg tablets

Dosages:
For muscle relaxation, 350 mg dose t.i.d (on short term basis)

3). Cyclobenzaprine
Availability: 10 mg tablets

Dosages:
For muscle relaxation, 10 mg dose t.i.d or q.i.d. (On Long-term basis)

4). Diazepam
Availability: 2, 5 and 10 mg tablets [3]

Dosages:
For muscle relaxation, 5-10 mg q.i.d. this must be used on short-term basis for not more than 2 weeks.

DENTAL CONSIDERATION:

- Monitor the vital signs of patient for having possible cardiovascular effects.
- Identify the need for use of CNS Muscle relaxants.
- Patient using it for backache should sit on dental chair with care and use anxiety reduction protocol to reduce anxiety level.
- Medicament for anxiety reduction include Valium (diazepam) 2-10 mg, or Ativan (Lorazepam) 1-4 mg or Xanax (alprazolam) 0.25-0.5 mg 30-60 minutes before the start of dental surgery.

- Patient diagnosed with MFPDS should have prescribed muscle relaxant adjunctive to NSAIDs or low-dose antidepressant and massage therapy.
- Advocate use of good oral hygiene with mechanical tooth brushing, dental flossing and with chemical medicament like Chlorhexidine mouth rinse.

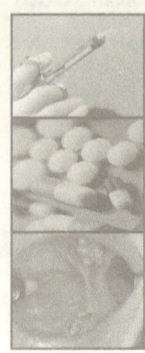

CHAPTER 25

Corticosteroids

Steroids are hormones synthesized by the adrenal cortex. There are two main groups' glucocorticoids and mineralocorticoids.

Glucocorticoids are essential for the utilization of carbohydrates, fats and proteins by the body and for normal response to stress. While *mineralocorticoids*, are necessary for the regulation of salt and water balance.

CLASSIFICATION:

Short-to medium acting:
> Hydrocortisone (Cortisol)
> Cortisone
> Prednisone
> Prednisolone
> Methylprednisolone
> Meprednisone

Intermediate acting:
> Triamcinolone
> Paramethasone

Long acting:
  Betamethasone
  Dexamethasone

MECHANISM OF ACTION: (PHYSIOLOGIC ACTION)

Synthesis and secretion: The major glucocorticoid in humans is cortisol. Cortisol gets synthesize from cholesterol by adrenal cortex (zona fasciculate and zona reticularis) and releases into circulation under the influence of ACTH.

In the circulation, 75% is bound to protein known as corticosteroid binding globulin (CBG). Twenty percent is circulating free while remaining 5% binds to albumin. Albumin has large capacity for storage bind but have low affinity for corticosteroids.

Mechanism of Action: cortisone has widely distributed receptors throughout the body cells exhibiting different functions on various cells. The genes are from 10-100 in cells that are influenced by corticosteroids however not all the genes are activated in each cells. Therefore, they show different responses in different cells of the body.

Free Corticosteroids bind to receptors on cell membrane know as 'heat shock proteins' of which hsp 90 is most common. The receptor steroid complex then moves intracellularly and binds in the nucleus does its action on DNA or RNA of the cell, creating mRNA, ultimately synthesize protein, and perform its respective function. [9]

Functions of Corticosteroids:

Metabolic function: Glucocorticoids stimulate the gluconeogenesis pathway in fasting state and diabetes. They also increase uptake of aminoacids by liver, kidney and increase the enzyme activity required for gluconeogenesis. They also increase glycogen deposition in the liver further adding pathway of gluconeogenesis (glucose synthesis from protein).

Lipids they inhibit uptake of glucose by the lipids leading to lipolysis. However, increase in insulin secretion in response to gluconeogenesis will lead to lipogenesis that ultimately lead to net increase in fat deposition.

In the fasting state adequate supply of glucose to the brain is via breakdown of protein from muscle catabolism, glucose form gluconeogenesis, inhibition of peripheral glucose uptake and stimulation of lipolysis.

Catabolic effect:

Catabolic effect of corticosteroids is on muscles, fat, connective tissue and skin. Catabolic effect in children may lead to inhibition of growth, and in Cushing syndrome lead to osteoporosis.

Anti-inflammatory effect:

Corticosteroids cause an increase in neutrophil concentration in circulation by two ways, 1. Increase influx of neutrophils from bone marrow into circulation, 2. Decrease migration from blood vessels ultimately decreasing the number of cells at inflammation site.

At the same time, they cause a decrease in T &B lymphocytes, monocytes, eosinophils and basophils via migrating them into the lymphoid tissue from the circulation.

They also reduce the synthesis of prostaglandins and leukotrienes from the activation of phospholipase A_2. They increase the concentration of lipocortins (member of the annexin family protein) which reduces the availability of phopholipid substrate of phopholipase A_2.

They inhibit the activity of kinins and bacterial endotoxin and histamine release from basophil cells leading to vasoconstriction and reducing capillary permeability.

Immunosuppressive effect:

Corticosteroids reduce the function of leukocytes and tissue macrophages. That is the phagocytising activity and killing of microorganism is reduced by reducing the production of interferon-gamma, interleukin-1 and TNF and plasminogen activator.

However, larger doses can reduce the production of antibodies but smaller doses like prednisone (20 mg/day) cannot affect its production.

Other effects:

Corticosteroids, its high doses and prolong use contribute to the development of peptic ulcer.

They suppress the release of ACTH, beta-lipoproteins, FSH and TSH.

On the development of fetus, corticosteroids (glucocorticoids) stimulate the production of surfactants. [3]

INDICATIONS:

Medical uses:

- For the diagnosis of Addison's disease; Short ACTH stimulation test, a tetracosactide (ACTH analogue) is given intramuscularly or intravenously. After 30 minutes of administration plasma cortisol level is measured. In normal individual cortisol, level is more than 600 nmol /litre. While in individuals with Addison's disease, have cortisol level below 400 nmol/litre. Cortisol level 400-600 nmol/L is on borderline.

- For the diagnosis of Cushing syndrome (in which there is excess secretion of ACTH from pituitary tumour) Dexamethasone suppression test, in which dexamethasone 1mg is given at midnight and the plasma cortisol level is suppressed the following morning in normal individual, while in cushing syndrome this suppression fails to occur because ACTH suppression has failed in response to dexamethasone injection.

- For Addison's disease: (in which adrenal cortex is destroyed leading to reduce production of glucocorticoids, mineralocorticoids and sex steroid production). Dosage;

hydrocortisone 20-30 mg daily, prednisolone 7.5 mg daily, fludrocortisone (mineralocorticoid) 50-300 µg daily. [9]

- <u>Allergic reactions:</u> Asthma, bee sting, contact dermatitis and drug reactions
- <u>Collagen vascular disorders:</u> giant cell arteritis, temporal arteritis, lupus erythematosus and PMR [9]
- <u>Gastrointestinal disease:</u> inflammatory bowel diseases, Crohn's disease and ulcerative colitis
- <u>Pulmonary diseases:</u> prevention of infant respiratory distress syndrome, bronchial asthma, COPD and sarcoidosis
- <u>Organ transplants:</u> prevention and treatment of rejection
- <u>Skin diseases:</u> atopic dermatitis, lichen planus, pemphigus.
- <u>Infections:</u> gram-negative septicaemia, occasionally helpful to suppress excessive inflammation.
- <u>Inflammatory conditions of bone and joints:</u> arthritis, bursitis and tenosynovitis

Dental uses:

- They are use in the treatment of unilateral headache due to temporal giant cell arteritis and/or PMR. [9]
- Topically use for oral lesions like RAS (recurrent Aphthous stomatitis/ulcers), lichen planus, and vesiculobullous diseases like pemphigus vulgaris, mucous membrane pemphigoid, and erythema multiforme and epidermolysis bullosa. [7]
- Topically use for oral lesions of sarcoidosis, and Crohn's disease. In addition, they are use systemically for these diseases.
- Triamcenolone injection has been successful into the lesion of oral submucous fibrosis.
- Use for desquamative gingivitis and dentine hypersensitivity. [4]
- In oral surgery, after the extraction of tooth to reduce inflammation and pain

- Use in dental office after the onset of allergy to L.A or any other medications or due to latex gloves use
- Use for TMJ arthritis symptoms.

SIDE EFFECTS:

Physiological:
Suppression of adrenal and/or pituitary hormone
Pathological:
Cardiovascular: increased blood pressure
Gastrointestinal: pancreatitis
Renal: polyuria, Nocturia
CNS: Depression, Euphoria, psychosis and insomnia
Bone and muscle: osteoporosis, proximal myopathy and wasting, aseptic necrosis of the hip and pathological fractures
Skin: thinning and easy bruising
Eyes: Cataracts
Increased susceptibility to infection: septicaemia, fungal infections, Reactivation of TB [9]

INDIVIDUAL DRUGS: [3]

1). Cortisone:
Availability: 5, 10, 25 mg tablets.

2). Hydrocortisone:
Availability: 5, 10, 20 mg tablets.

3). Hydrocortisone acetate:
Availability: 25, 50 mg /ml
Use for intralesional, soft-tissue or intra-articular injection.

4). Hydrocortisone sodium succinate:
Availability: 100, 250 mg /vial for IV or IM injections.

5). Methylprednisolone:
Availability: 2, 4, 8, 16 mg tablets.

6). Prednisolone:
Availability: 5 mg tablet.

7). Prednisolone acetate:
Availability: 25, 50 mg/ml for soft-tissue and intra-articular injection

8). Triamcinolone:
Availability: 1, 2, 4, 8 mg tablets.

9). Triamcinolone hexacetonide:
Availability 5, 20 mg/ml for intra-articular, intralesional or sub-lesional injection

DENTAL CONSIDERATION:

- Identify the cause for taking Corticosteroids.
- Prepare the patient for dental surgery according to surgical guidelines on corticosteroids.
- Give premedication hydrocortisone 100 mg (IM), then do surgery and resume to normal dose after the surgery immediately if no complication and eating normally.
- Alternatively, give premedication of hydrocortisone 100 mg IM, then during surgery maintain 20 mg orally 6 hourly or 50 mg IM, every 6 hours for 24 hours if not eating. Then resumption of normal dose after 24 hours if no complication occurs. [9]
- Prolong use of corticosteroids can predispose patient to oral candidiasis. Check for its signs. Oral inhaler or nasal spray can put the patient at risk for oral and oropharyngeal candidiasis respectively.

- Prolong use of corticosteroids may also mask oral signs of diseases so assess and monitor these signs.
- Corticosteroid may also cause immunosuppresion, delay in healing and mask signs of infection. So give prophylactic antibiotics before commencing any dental procedure.
- Dry mouth due to corticosteroid use may predispose patient to dental caries, periodontal disease and candidiasis. So manage dry mouth with tart, sugar free chewing gum, and/ or saliva substitute.
- Avoid prescribing aspirin containing drugs.
- Patient on chronic corticosteroids use may also develop blood dyscrasias (sign and symptoms are fever, severe sore throat, bleedings and poor wound healing). Patient with such symptoms should be referred to medical specialist and then manage accordingly. [10]

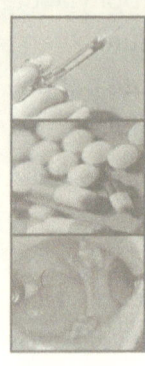

CHAPTER 26
Anti-Diabetics

CLASSIFICATION:

Sulfonylurea:
- Tolbutamide
- Tolazamide
- Glibenclamide
- Glimepiride
- Glipizide
- Chlorpropamide

Biguanides:
- Metformin
- Buformin
- Phenformin

Thiazolidinedione Derivatives:
- Pioglitazone
- Rosiglitazone
- Troglitazone

Aldose reductase inhibitors:

Tolrestat

Epalrestat

Ranirestat

Fidarestat

MODE AND MECHANISM OF ACTION:

I.   Sulfonylureas: they are insulin secretogagues in the sense that they act on the beta cells of the pancreas (they are ineffective in individuals having no or impaired functional beta cell mass) blocking ATP-sensitive potassium channels and blocks potassium efflux. Which results in depolarization leading to calcium influxultimately secreting insulin. (Note: insulin secretion is enhanced in response to the following agents: glucose, mannose, leucine, vagal stimulation, and sulfonylurea).

II. Biguanides: they are considered to be insulin sensitizer yet they donot promote insulin secretion. They activates the enzyme AMP-Kinase, which is involved in GLUT-4 metabolism and fatty acid oxidation but its mechanism of action remains unclear at cellular level. They also reduce gluconeogenesis resulting in reduce hepatic glucose output. (Note: GLUT-4 is a glucose transport protein that enables peripheral cells like muscle and adipose tissues to uptake glucose inside the cells in response to insulin binding to its receptor on respective peripheral cells)

III. Thiazolidinediones: they are also insulin sensitizer like Biguanides; they bind to nuclear receptor (PPAR-gamma) *peroxisome proliferator activated receptor gamma*, which regulate genes responsible for insulin action and lipid metabolism. Thiazolidinediones lower circulating insulin level relative to plasma glucose but donot return glucose level to normal. They potentiate the effect of injected or endogenous insulin. So they are use alone or in combination with other drugs like injected insulin or insulin secretogagues.

IV. Aldose reductase inhibitors: aldose reductase is an enzyme this is present in those cells in the human body, which are not sensitive to insulin (like lenses, peripheral nerves and glomerulus). They catalyze one of the steps in polyol pathway (sorbitol) which metabolize glucose to form sorbitol and fructose. The sorbitol accumulates in these non-insulin sensitive tissues causing damage to them. Like eyes (retinopathy), nerves (neuropathy) and glomerulus (nephropathy). (Note: excess glucose is metabolized in the lenses by aldose reductase to form alcohol; the lenses are impermeable to the alcohol hence it imbibes water in the lens leading to diabetic cataract).

Therefore, aldose reductase inhibitors are a class of dugs being studied as a way to prevent eye and nerve damage in diabetic patients.

INDICATIONS:

- Sulfonylureas are drugs use for NIDD, in those patients whose beta cell mass is functionally normal. It is avoided in diabetic overweight patients. Tolbutamide is the safest drug in the very elderly because of its short duration of action.
- Metformin does not predispose to weight gain so it is particularly useful in patients who are overweight. It has also proved unexpectedly beneficial to reduce cardiovascular risk in diabetes. [2]

ADVERSE EFFECTS:

- Hypoglycaemia
- Weight gain and hyperinsulinemia

- They should be use with caution in Patient with hepatic and renal insufficiency because its slow excretion may induce hypoglycaemia.
- GI: vomiting, nausea and diarrhoea
- Lactic acidosis in CHF and megaloblastic anaemia (Biguanides)
- Women taking contraceptives and Thiazolidinediones may become pregnant.
- Weight gain, headache and anaemia (particular to Thiazolidinediones)

INDIVIDUAL DRUGS:

1. **Tolbutamide:**
   Availability: 500 mg tablets
   Dosage: initial dose 1-2 g daily
   Maintenance dose: 250-1000 mg daily

2. **Glimepiride:**
   Availability: 1 mg, 2 mg and 4 mg tablets
   Dosage: initial dose: 1-2 mg orally O.D
   Maintenance dose: 1-4 mg O.D maximum upto 8 mg per day.

3. **Metformin:**
   Availability: 500 mg tablets
   Dosage: 500 mg orally b.i.d (with morning and evening meal)

Drug-Drug interactions:

H_2—antagonist: increase hypoglycaemic effect of oral antidiabetic drugs.

NSAIDs: increase hypoglycaemic effect of oral anti-diabetics drugs.

Salicylates: increase hypoglycaemic effect by decreasing plasma protein binding.

Sulphonamides: increase hypoglycaemic effect by decreasing plasma protein binding.

Sympathomimetics: increase requirements for sulfonylurea.

Tricyclic antidepressants: increase hypoglycaemic effect of oral anti-diabetics. [10]

INSULIN

CLASSIFICATION:

Insulin aspart
Insulin detemir
Insulin glargine
Insulin lispro
Insulin glulisine
NPH insulin suspension
Regular insulin [2]

MODE OF ACTION:

Insulin is a polypeptide hormone that has two peptide chains connected to each other by disulfide bonds. They are formed as precursor known as pro-insulin. This pro-insulin undergoes a proteolytic cleavage to form insulin and C-peptide. Circulating C-peptide is a measure of index for insulin level. Insulin secretion is mediated by many agents including blood glucose many other amino acids, hormones and autonomic mediators.

Amplifiers of glucose-induced insulin release are:

I.   *Enteric hormones*
     Glucagon like peptide

Gastrin inhibitory peptide
Cholecystokinin
Secretin, gastrin

II. *Neural amplifiers*
Beta-adrenoceptor stimulation

III. *Amino acids*
Arginine

Inhibitors of insulin release are:

IV. *Neural:*
Alpha-sympathetic effect of catecholamine

V. *Humoral:*
Somatostatin

VI. *Drugs:*
Diazoxide, phenytoin, colchicine [1]

Rapid-acting and short-acting insulin:

(Insulin aspart, insulin lispro, regular insulin and insulin glulisine)
Peak level of insulin lispro is 30-90 minutes of injection, while that of regular insulin is 50-120 minutes. *Duration of action of short-acting is upto 6-8hours.* They are administered with a meal to mimic the action of prandial insulin secretion. Mostly they are administered 15 minutes before meal or after a meal. They are also use concomitantly with longer-acting insulin.

Intermediate-acting insulin:

(NPH insulin or insulin isophane)

It is used in conjunction with positively charged polypeptide protamine, which forms a less soluble complex. That is why they are classified as intermediate-acting insulin. Their *duration of action is upto 18 hours*. They are only use subcutaneously and for all kind of diabetes but not for emergency diabetes (ketoacidosis).

Long-acting insulin:

(Insulin glargine and insulin detemir)

Insulin detemir has fatty acid chain, which is associated with albumin protein as a result slow dissociation from albumin makes it *long-acting (upto 24 hours)*.

SIDE EFFECTS:

- Hypoglycaemia, symptoms include

  a. Tachycardia
  b. Vertigo
  c. Diaphoresis (excessive sweating)
  d. Confusion

- At the site of injection (swelling, stinging, itching, warmth and redness)
- Hypersensitivity (urticaria, angioedema, bulla, anaphylaxis)

Drug-Drugs Interactions:

Corticosteroids: decrease effect of insulin because of hyperglycaemic effect of steroids.

Epinephrine: decrease effect of insulin because of epinephrine induced hyperglycaemia.

Phenytoin: phenytoin induces hyperglycaemia leading to decrease diabetic control.

Salicylates: increase hypoglycaemic effect of insulin.

Tetracycline: may increase hypoglycaemic effect of insulin.

DENTAL CONSIDERATION:

- Obtain medical history from the patient.
- Ask for whether patient is on oral antidiabetic drugs or on insulin.
- Schedule an early morning appointment for anxious patient and reduce the waiting room sitting time.
- Dentist may go for anxiety reduction protocol in case the patient is very anxious. That is valium (diazepam) 2-10 mg or ativan (lorazepam) 1-4 mg or xanax (alprazolam) 0.25-0.5 mg, all drugs be taken 1 hour before commencing dental surgery.
- Before going for dental surgery, ask the patient to check blood glucose level including the test of glycosylated Haemoglobin (Hb_{A1}-C). Ideally, it should be less than 7% otherwise 8% is also optimal. [9]
- Keep sugar candy or fruit juice with you while doing dental operation for diabetic patient, for he or she may go into hypoglycaemia due to anxiety or already taken hypoglycaemic agents.
- Prescribe also prophylactic antibiotics, for diabetic patient is highly susceptible to infection after dental surgery or deep scaling.
- Give frequent appointments in order to check for extraction site healing as diabetes may delay healing.
- Diabetic patient experiences dry mouth, which makes him susceptible to dental caries, periodontal diseases and candidal infection.
- So advice, fluoride home treatment with use of alcohol free mouth rinses.

- Studies have revealed that diabetes and periodontal diseases are mutually synergistic to one another. That is if patient has gingivitis and/or periodontitis with heavy calculus deposits it will aggravate the patient diabetic condition and like wise diabetes will aggravate the patient's periodontal diseases.

- Therefore, frequent check up by periodontologist is mandatory in order to keep both diabetic and periodontal conditions in control.

ANTI-ALLERGIC

Anti-allergic are those drugs, which are used to counteract the effects of allergies. They include 'Anti-histamine drugs' and other drugs used as prophylaxis for allergies like 'Mast-cell degranulation inhibitors' and 'Leukotriene inhibitors'.

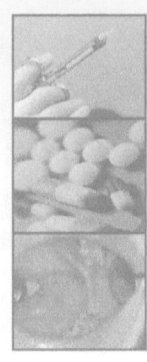

CHAPTER 27

Anti-Histamines (H1 Anti-histamines)

CLASSIFICATION:

First generation:

Ethanolamines: Piperazines:

Diphenhydramine Hydroxyzine

Dimenhydrinate Cyclizine

Doxylamine Meclizine

Alkylamines: Phenothaizine:

Brompheniramine Promethazine

Chlorpheniramine

Second generation:

Piperadines:

Fexofenadine

Terfenadine

Astemizole

Miscellaneous:
    Loratadine
    Desloratadine
    Ceterizine
    Levocetirizine
    Acrivastine

MODE OF ACTION:

Occurrence:

Histamine is present widely in the human tissues with more abundance in lungs, skin and gastrointestinal track. When histamine is released from mast cells, basophils, CNS neurons and gastric mucosa parietal cells, they bind to four receptors known as H_1, H_2, H_3, and H_4
    Among them as H_1 and H_2 are of much clinical importance.

Action:

They exhibit the following actions on the these sites;
Bronchial smooth muscle:
Constricition of Bronchial smooth muscles result in symptoms of asthma.
    Intestinal smooth muscle:
Constrictions of intestinal smooth muscles lead to muscle cramps and diarrhoea.
    Exocrine excretion:
Increase production of nasal and mucosal secretion leading to respiratory symptoms.
    Skin:
Dilatation and increased permeability of capillaries result in protein leakage and fluid into the tissue. Signs include "wheal formation", "reddening" due to vasodilation and "flare".

H_1 blockers qualitatively block histamine receptors thus inhibiting the action of histamine on it. [2]

INDICATIONS:

Allergy:

They are the drug of choice for allergic rhinitis and urticaria. However, not for asthma because histamine is only one of the mediators that is released along with other mediators (Leukotrienes are the main mediators in asthma).

Anti emetic:

As they also block central H_1 and muscarinic receptors, they are effective in treating motion sickness and nausea.

Somnifecients:

They are also be used to treat insomnia as they cross blood-brain barrier to induce sedation.

SIDE EFFECTS:

Oral:

Dry mouth

Nose:

Dry nasal mucosa

Eye:

Blurred vision

CNS:

Sedation, tinnitus, fatigue, dizziness, tremors and vertigo

CVS:

Tachycardia and hypotension

Genitourinary:

Urinary retention and erectile dysfunction [10]

Drug-Drug interactions:

Tricyclic-antidepressants: have additive anticholinergic effect with anti-histamine drugs.

Benzodiazepine, barbiturates, narcotics and phenothiazines: Their concomitant use with anti-histamine drugs may lead to drowsiness, stupor, lethargy, respiratory depression, coma and possibly death.

INDIVIDUAL DRUGS:

1) **Diphenhydramine:**
   Availability: 25 mg capsule
   Dosage: 25-50 mg dose every q.i.d

2) **Chlorpheniramine:**
   Availability: 4 mg, 8 mg tablets
   Dosage: 4 mg every 4-6 hours

3) **Brompheniramine:**
   Availability: 4, 12 mg tablets
   Dosage: 4 mg every 4-6 hours

4) **Promethazine:**
   Availability: 12.5, 25 mg tablets
   Dosage; 12.5-25 mg once daily

5) **Cetirizine:**
   Availability: 5, 10 mg tablets
   Dosage: 5-10 mg once daily

6) **loratadine:**
   Availability: 10 mg tablets
   Dosage: 10 mg once daily

7) **Fexofenadine**
   Availability: 60, 120 mg tablets. [3]
   Dosage: 60-120 mg once daily

LEUKOTRIENE INHIBITORS:

Leukotrienes have been strongly implicated in the pathogenesis of inflammation especially in chronic diseases such as asthma and inflammatory bowel disease. The peptide leukotrienes particularly LTC_4 and LTD_4 are potent broncho-constrictors and cause an increase in micro-vascular permeability, plasma exudation and mucus secretion in the airway. High and low, affinity LTD_4 receptors are present in the human lung tissue.

CLASSIFICATION:

Montelukast
Zafirlukast
Zileuton [2]

MECHANISM OF ACTION:

Leukotriene inhibitors act by two ways.

1). Inhibition of 5-lipooxygenase pathway: by which they prevent leukotriene synthesis.
2). Inhibition of binding of leukotriene D_4 to its receptor on target tissues thereby, preventing its action.

INDICAITONS:

They are use as a prophylaxis for asthma and allergic rhinitis (hay fever).

ADVERSE EFFECTS:

- Eosiniphilic vasculitis (Chug-Strauss syndrome)
- Headache
- Dyspepsia
- Elevation in serum hepatic enzymes

INDIVIDUAL DRUGS:

Montelukast:

It is LTD_4 receptor antagonist.
They are orally taken once daily.
Availability: 10 mg tablets, 4 mg chewable tablets.
Dosage: 10 mg per day 1-2 months before the start of a season

MAST CELL DEGRANULATION INHIBITORS

CLASSIFICATION:

Cromolyn
Nedocromil

MECHANISM OF ACTION:

They alter chloride channel function of mast cells after the cells are sensitized by the antigen-antibody reaction. The rupture and degranulation of mast cell is inhibited. Recently it has been found that these drugs also inhibit the function of other cells (involved in late inflammatory response).

INDICATIONS:

As a prophylaxis for asthma and allergic rhinitis

They are not effective against acute attack.

They are drugs of choice in young children for asthma and hay fever.

SIDE EFFECTS:

- Cough,
- Bitter taste
- Irritation of larynx and pharynx
- Toxic reactions are rare.

INDIVIDUAL DRUGS:

Cromolyn sodium:

Availability: Pulmonary aerosol 800 microgram /puff in 200 dose container, 20 mg capsule for inhalation.

Nasal aerosol; 5.2 mg/puff [3]

DENTAL CONSIDERATION:

- Ask for the reason of taking anti-histamine drugs.
- Patient with allergic rhinitis and asthma may need to sit on dental chair in semi-supine position.
- If patient has frequent attack of status asthmaticus then either defer dental procedure and take a consult from patient's primary care physician. [8]
- Alternatively, take necessary precautions like keeping pre-loaded epinephrine, pre-loaded beta agonist inhalers (Ventolin and Steroids) while doing dental operation.
- Anti-histamine drugs cause dry mouth, which predisposes the patient to dental caries, periodontal disease and candidiasis.
- Treat dry mouth with tart, sugar free chewing gum (xylitol) and/ or saliva substitute.

- Patient may also take frequent sips of water to counteract the effect of xerostomia and dysphagia (difficulty in swallowing) during eating.
- Advocate fluoride home treatment.
- Prescribe Chlorhexidine mouthwash for oral rinse twice daily.
- Avoid prescribing alcohol containing mouth rinse.

ANTI-MICROBIAL

Antibiotics are the substance produced by or derived from the microorganism that destroys or inhibits the growth of other microorganisms. Antibiotics are use to treat infections caused by organisms that are sensitive to them, usually bacteria or fungi. They may alter normal microbial content of the body by destroying one or more groups of harmless or beneficial organisms, which may result in infection due to overgrowth of resistant organisms.

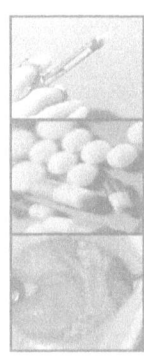

CHAPTER 28

PENICILLINS

CLASSIFICATION:

Amoxicillin
Ampicillin
Methicillin
Dicloxacillin
Oxacillin
Piperacillin
Penicillin G
Penicllin V

MODE OF ACTION:

Penicillin is from the bactericidal group of antibiotics. They are beta-lactams as they contain beta-lactam ring attach to thiazolidine ring in their structure. They are highly efficient against proliferating bacteria, those bacteria that are involved in the synthesis of their cell wall. Bacteria has penicillin binding protein PBP (an enzyme involved in the synthesis of cell wall, PBP catalyzes the transpeptidase reaction that removes the terminal alanine making cross-link with nearby peptide). Penicillin binds to this enzyme PBP hindering it from making cross-links between their peptidoglycan chains.

Resistance to penicillin:

Resistance to this class of drug occurs in three ways

I. <u>By inactivation of antibiotic by beta lactamase (enzyme produce by bacteria),</u> beta lactamase is produce by Staphylococcus aureus, Haemophilus and E.coli which hydrolyze only penicillin. Whereas beta lactamase produce by Pseudomonas aeruginosa and Enterobacter also hydrolyze cephalosporin along with Penicllin.

II. <u>By permeability barrier that prevents entry of antibiotic into the cell.</u> This barrier is mostly present in Gram-negative bacteria, but not in Gram-positive bacteria.

III. <u>By conformational changes in PBP structure</u> PBP structure produce by staphylococci and pneumococci have low affinity for binding to beta-lactam antibiotics. This lead to the production of an organism known as MRSA (methicillin resistance staphylococcus aureus). [2]

INDICATIONS:

- Use for bone and joint infections including TMJ (caused by staphylococcus aureus). [8]
- Use for skin and soft tissue infection as in maxillofacial surgery and intra-oral surgical procedure (caused by streptococcus pyogenes and/or staphylococcus aureus).
- Use for Pharyngitis (caused by streptococcus pyogenes).
- Use for Endocarditis (caused by streptococcus viridans secondary to dental extraction or by enterococcus faecalis). [7]

SIDE EFFECTS:

Most common side effect to penicillin is hypersensitivity which may range form skin rashes and fever to anaphylactic shock.

Hematologic problem may occur such as in those patients who are already on anti-coagulants or having a disease, which predisposes them to bleeding.

There may also be GI disturbance due to altering the normal gut flora.

It may also cause supra infection in GIT leading to pseudomembranous colitis (caused by clostridium difficile).

They may also provoke seizure in patients who are at risk for epileptic attack. [10]

INDIVIDUAL DRUGS:

1. **Amoxicillin:**
   Availability: 250 and 500 mg capsules
   Dosage: 500 mg dose t.i.d for 5-7 days

2. **Amoxicillin /potassium Clavulanate**
   Availability: 375 mg, 625 mg and 1g tablets
   Dosage: 375 mg or 625 mg t.i.d, or 1g b.i.d for 5-7 days

3. **Penicillin G:**
   Availability: (oral) 0.2, 0.25, 0.4, 0.8 million unit tablets
   (Parenteral) 1,2 3, 5, 10, 20 million units.
   Dosage: IV 1-4 mU every 4-6 hours

DENTAL CONSIDERATION:

- Check for any signs or symptoms of allergy when penicillin is administered.

- If patient's response is allergic immediately, withdraw the drug.
- Signs and symptoms of allergy may include skin rashes, angioneuretic oedema, intense itching, fever, joint swelling and respiratory distress.
- Patient with asthma, hay fever, urticaria and those allergic to cephalosporin are more predisposed to show allergic reactions with penicillin.
- Complete the entire antibiotic course, for incomplete therapy will bring resistance to the patient with many organisms.
- For prevention of infective endocarditis penicillin are taken 30 minutes (in case of parenteral route of administration) before or 1 hour (in case of oral administration) before the start of dental procedure.
- The dose of penicillin as a prophylaxis to infective endocarditis is Amoxicillin Adults: 2 g, Children: 50mg/kg orally 1 hour before procedure.
- Alternative to Amoxicillin is Ampicillin Adults: 2.0 g IM or IV, Children: 50mg/kg IM or IV within 30 minutes before procedure.
- Super infection with penicillin may include furry tongue, diarrhoea and vaginal or rectal itching.
- For streptococcal infection, which may lead to complications like glomerulunephritis and/or rheumatic fever, the dose should be taken for minimum of 14 days in order to prevent these complications.

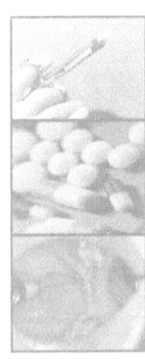

CHAPTER 29

Cephalosporins

CLASSIFICATION:

First generation cephalosporin
  Cefradine
  Cefalexin
  Cefadroxil
  Cefazolin

Second-generation cephalosporin
  Cefuroxime
  Cefaclor
  Cefoxitin

Third generation cephalosporin
  Cefotaxime
  Ceftazidime
  Cefixime
  Cefpodoxime
  Ceftriaxone
  Cefdinir

<u>Fourth generation cephalosporin</u>
Cefepime [2]

INDICATIONS:

Cephalosporins are the most effective treatment for sinusitis.

They are use for urinary tract infection, cellulitis and other soft tissues infection caused by streptococcus and staphylococcus organisms.

They are use for biliary track infection.

They are use for pneumonia and septicaemia.

Second generation Cephalosporin is also effective against bacteriodes (anaerobic organisms).

Third generation Cephalosporin is also effective against meningitis.

ADVERSE EFFECTS:

- Patients who are allergic to penicillin are also more likely to suffer allergic reaction from cephalosporin.
- They may cause hematologic toxicity (bleeding and poor wound healing).
- Disulfiram like reaction may also occur with them.
- When used with diuretic it may be nephrotoxic.
- Super infection may also occur, caused by fungi, MRSA, and enterococci. [2]

INDIVIDUAL DRUGS:

1. **Cefadroxil:**
   Availability: 500 mg capsules, 1g tablets.
   Dosage: 0.5-1 g dose b.i.d

2. **Cefoxitin:**
   Availability: (parenterally) 1,2, 10 g per vial.
   Dosage: 1-2 g dose every 6-8 hours.

3. **Cefuroxime:**
   Availability: 125, 250 and 500 mg tablets.
   Dosage: 0.75-1.5 g dose t.i.d

4. **Ceftriaxone:**
   Availability: (parenteral) 0.25, 0.5, 1, 2, and 10 g per vial) [3]
   Dosage: IV 1-4 g O.D

DENTAL CONSIDERATION:

- Check for any signs or symptoms of allergy when cephalosporin is administered.
- If patient's response is allergic immediately, withdraw the drug.
- Signs and symptoms of allergy may include skin rashes, angioneuretic oedema, intense itching, fever, joint swelling and respiratory distress.
- Patient with asthma, hay fever, urticaria and those allergic to Penicillin are more susceptible to show allergic reactions to Cephalosporin.
- Complete the entire antibiotic course, for incomplete therapy will bring resistance to the patient with many organisms.
- For prevention of infective endocarditis, Cephalosporin is taken 1 hour (in case of oral administration) before the start of dental procedure.
- The doses of Cephalosporin for the prophylaxis of infective endocarditis is, cefalexin or cefadroxil—Adults: 2 g, Children: 50mg/kg orally 1 hour before procedure. [5]

- Super-infection with cephalosporin may include furry tongue, diarrhoea and vaginal or rectal itching. This may be treated with topical Nystatin application.
- Avoid alcohol and alcohol containing mouth rinses as disulfiram-like reaction may occur with Cephalosporin.
- Yogurt or buttermilk can be prescribed for abdominal diarrhoea related to intestinal super infection because they may help to normalize the gut flora.
- Oral medication of cephalosporin is preferably taken on empty stomach to avoid binding with food.
- Lower dose of cephalosporin should be administered to patient with renal impairment.

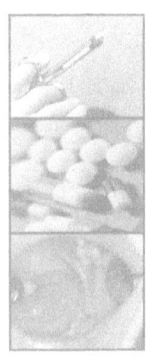

CHAPTER 30

Tetracyclines

CLASSIFICATION:

Tetracycline
Oxytetracycline
Doxycycline
Demeclocycline
Lymecycline
Minocycline

MODE OF ACTION:

They are bacteriostatic as they are the major protein synthesis inhibitor. These drugs enter into bacteria cell by passive diffusion and by energy-dependant (active diffusion) transport protein mechanism. They compete with tRNA for the 'A' site on ribosome. Hence, the binding of tRNA to mRNA-ribosome complex is inhibited, which ultimately inhibit protein synthesis. [2]

INDICATIONS:

As they are broad-spectrum anti-biotics, they cover Gram-positive and Gram-negative bacteria. However, it has also shown widespread resistance so its use has declined. Nevertheless, the resistance with respiratory infections has receded with decrease use. So again, it is the drug of choice for respiratory infections.

- It is use for respiratory infection like excacerbation of chronic bronchitis and community acquired pneumonia.
- It is use for chlamydial infection like non-gonococcal urethritis lymphogranuloma venereum and pelvic inflammatory diseases (caused by Chlamydia trachomatis). In addition, it is useful for psittacosis (caused by Chlamydia psittaci).
- It is use for Lyme disease (caused by Borellia burgdorgferi) signs and symptoms include skin lesions, headache and fever followed by meningo-encephalitis and arthritis.

Dental uses:

- Treatment of certain periodontal diseases like Localized juvenile periodontitis and Refractory periodontitis.
- Doxycycline 10% gel has been approved by FDA, as a local injection (syringe atridox) into the periodontal pocket
- SDD (sub-therapeutic dose doxycycline) is used in 20 mg dose b.i.d as a host-modulating agent for the improvement of gingival pocket attachment and bone loss. This dose is too low to act as antibiotic. The duration of course is from 3-9 months. (20 mg dose exert its effect by enzymes, cytokines and osteoclast inhibition rather than any antibiotic effect). [4]

SIDE EFFECTS:

Commonest side effect includes GI disturbances caused by irritation and modification of gut flora.

They are deposited in bones and teeth as they chelate Calcium ions therefore they cause discoloration of teeth and get deposit in bones leading to bone deformities. (Discoloration includes enamel and dentinal hypoplasia, dark brownish discoloration).

Therefore, they are contra-indicated in children upto 8 years of age, pregnant women and nursing mothers.

Phototoxicity also has been reported with the use of tetracyclines.

Superinfection has also occurred such as overgrowth of candida (candidiasis) and Pseuodomembranous colitis (by clostridium difficile). [2]

INDIVIDUAL DRUGS:

1. **Tetracycline:**
   Availability: 100, 250 mg capsules, 250, 500 mg tablets.
   Dosage: For refractory periodontitis, 250 mg dose q.i.d for 10 days

2. **Doxycycline:**
   Availability: 50, 100 mg tablets and capsules.
   Dosage: For chronic periodontitis, loading dose 200 mg (100 mg b.i.d) on first day followed by maintenance dose of 100 mg O.D for 14 days
   Sub-therapeutic dose Doxycycline (SDD) includes 20 mg tablets b.i.d for minimum of 3 months and maximum of 9 months.

3. **Minocycline:**

   (It suppresses spirochetes and motile rods as effective as scaling and root planning from the gingival sulcus).

   It causes less phototoxicity and renal toxicity but may cause reversible vertigo. Moreover, it completely eliminates spirochetes for upto 2 months and improves whole of the periodontium.

   Availability: 50, 100 mg tablets and capsules.

   Dosage: 100 mg b.i.d for adult periodontitis

   Other preparations available for periodontal uses: [4]

4. **Minocycline microspheres (2%)**

   Dosage form: biodegradable powder in syringe

5. **Doxycycline gel (10%)**

   Dosage form: biodegradable mixture in syringe

DENTAL CONSIDERATION:

- Determine the reason for taking tetracycline as antibiotic.
- If the patient is pregnant then document the trimester.
- Take on full stomach to enhance absorption but donot take with milk, yogurt, cheese, ice cream, or other foods and drugs containing Calcium ions as it may precipitate calcium ions leading to deposition in bones and teeth.
- Zinc containing drugs, food and vitamins preparations should be avoided as it may interfere with drug absorption.
- Zinc containing food includes oyster, cooked lobster, dry oat flakes, liver and steamed crabs.
- Document the side effects such as sore throat, dysphagia, dizziness, hoarseness, fever, inflammation of mucous membranes and superinfection by Candida.
- Wear glasses to the patient as dental light may cause severe photosensitivity like that of sun.

- Tetracycline may cause tooth discoloration from third trimester upto 8 years of age. So avoid using during this period because it causes pigmentation of enamel and dentine.
- Use tetracycline 1 hour before or 2 hours after using an air-polishing device such as prophy jet. [10]

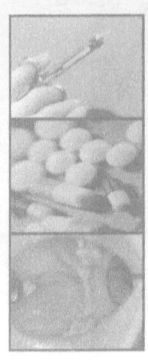

CHAPTER 31
Macrolides

CLASSIFICATION:

Erythromycin
Clarithromycin
Azithromycin
Spiramycin
Telithromycin

MODE OF ACTION:

They are bactericidal/ bacteriostatic. They irreversibly bind to ribosome (50 S) subunit thus hindering translocation step in protein synthesis. That is, the movement of tRNA from 'P' site to 'A' site is translocation, which is inhibited.

INDICATIONS:

Their anti-microbial spectrum is similar to that of penicillin. Erythromycin is effective against Gram-positive and spirochetes while Azithromycin is more effective against H.influenze, moxella and legionella.

So they are used as:

- (Erythromycin) In those patients who are allergic to penicillin.
- (Azithromycin) as they are more effective against H.influenze and moxella catarrhalis they are use in respiratory infections.
- (Azithromycin) is also use in urethritis caused by Chlamydia trachomatis.

Dental Uses:

- (Spiramycin) as it is secreted in saliva so it is used as an adjunctive therapy for periodontal diseases.
- (Azithromycin) is effective against gram-negative bacilli and anaerobes. Their concentration is 100-200 times higher in periodontal lesion than that of normal gingiva. As they penetrate into Fibroblasts and Phagocytes, they are actively transported to the site of inflammation when Phagocytes rupture during phagocytosis. [4]

SIDE EFFECTS:

GI disturbance is common to macrolides.

Hypersensitivity reactions have also been reported; including skin rashes, fever and transient hearing disturbances.

Cholestatic jaundice is also, the side effect been observed.

Opportunistic infection of vagina and GI track has also been reported. [2]

INDIVIDUAL DRUGS:

1. Azithromycin:

Availability: 250 mg capsules.

Dosage: initial loading dose is 500 mg on 1st day followed by maintenance dose of 250 mg O.D for next 4 days.

2. Clarithromycin:

Availability: 250, 500 mg tablets.

Dosage: For tonsillitis, pharyngitis and bronchitis; dose of 250 mg b.i.d for 7-14 days.

For duodenal ulcer associated with H.pylori infection 500 mg t.i.d for 2 weeks adjunctive to Omeprazole 40 mg.

3. Erythromycin:

Availability: 250, 500 mg tablets. [3]

Dosage: For respiratory infection, due to Mycoplasma pneumoniea, dose of 500 mg q.i.d for 5-10 days.

For intestinal amoebiasis, due to Entamoeba histolytica, dose of 250 mg q.i.d for 10-14 days.

DENTAL CONSIDERATION:

- Continue entire prescription without any interval, even signs and symptoms subside.
- Take on empty stomach to make it more effectively absorbed.
- Azithromycin is the drug of choice for many periodontal diseases due to its potent effect on gingival sulcus.
- It is also use as an alternative to penicillin and can be used in diabetic patients for improved healing of gingivitis and/or periodontitis. [10]

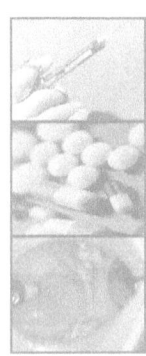

CHAPTER 32

Clindamycin

Clindamycin is effective against Gram-positive cocci and anaerobic bacteria including Bacteroides fragilis.

It is use as an alternative to penicillin and metronidazole in dental practice. As it covers anti-microbial spectrum of penicillin as well as metronidazole, so instead of using two drugs, one drug is a safe alternative.

MECHANISM OF ACTION:

Its mechanism of action is similar to that of macrolides.

INDICATIONS:

Its uses include staphylococcal infection of bones and joints including (TMJs) [8] and staphylococcal infection of eye (conjunctivitis).

SIDE EFFECTS:

Commonest side effect includes Pseudo-membranous colitis caused by clostridium difficile for, which the treatment is again Metronidazole.[2]

Availability: 75, 150, 300 mg capsules. [3]

Dosage:

As a prophylaxis for bacteria endocarditis 600 mg 1 hour prior to procedure or 600 mg, IV within 30 minutes before the start of dental procedure (dilutes and inject slowly).

For dental infections like peri-apical periodontitis, gingivitis, primary periodontitis and cellulitis, loading dose is 600 mg on first day followed by 300 mg maintenance dose q.i.d for next 3 days.

ANTI-PROTOZOA

Protozoa are motile, unicellular eukaryotic organism whose metabolism is much similar to that of human cells. Therefore, drugs used for the treatment of infections caused by these protozoa also affect human cells particularly those with high metabolic rate e-g neuronal cells, intestinal mucosal cells, renal tubular and bone marrow stem cells, protozoa includes amoeba, flagellates, sporozoa and ciliates.

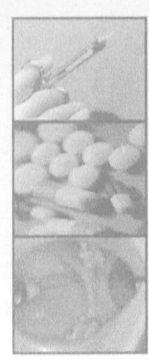

CHAPTER 33

Amoebicidal Drugs

CLASSIFICATION:

Metronidazole
Diloxanide
Tinidazole [1]

LIFE CYCLE OF ENTAMOEBA HISTOLYTICA:

It exists in cyst form outside the human body associated with faeces. When humans ingest faeces-contaminated food, the cyst is also ingested into intestinal lumen where they rupture and form trophozites. Trophozites are harmful when they penetrate intestinal mucosal cells because they ulcerate them (symptoms include bloody diarrhoea and abdominal pain), moreover; they are also fed by intestinal flora (bacteria). Therefore, after ulceration they may penetrate into systemic circulation and reach the liver. Here in the liver they cause amoebic liver abscess. The trophozite then slowly pass into the rectum and gets convert into cyst again where they are excreted along with the faeces hence life cycle completes.

Amebiasis may occur in two forms. One is symptomatic and other is asymptomatic. Therefore, in acute phase (symptomatic) drug of choice is metronidazole while for chronic phase (asymptomatic) drug of choice is Diloxanide.

(Note: antibiotic such as *tetracycline* or *paromomycin* is also added to the treatment regimen in order to kill intestinal flora hence eliminating primary source of food for Entamoeba histolytica).

METRONIDAZOLE:

It is a mixed Amoebicidal drug (i-e it has both luminal and systemic activity against E.histolytica).

MODE OF ACTION:

Metronidazole has nitro compound, which is an electron acceptor by which it binds to nucleus and protein of amoeba cell leading to cell death.

Metronidazole is also effective against anaerobic bacteria such as anaerobic cocci and Gram-negative bacilli (like Bacteroides fragilis) and anaerobic Gram-positive bacillus (Clostridium difficile).

INDICATIONS:

- It is use for Amoebic dysentery with or without antibiotic (e-g tetracycline).
- It is also use for Giardiasis caused by Giardia lamblia.
- It is a treatment of choice for pseudomembranous caused by Clostridium difficile. [1]

Dental uses include all those conditions in which there is high chance of anaerobic infections like [4]

- Chronic peri-apical abscess

- Cellulitis
- Post-operative dental surgery and/or Maxillo-facial surgery
- Advanced care adult periodontitis.
- Localized juvenile periodontitis (along with amoxicillin)
- Rapidly progressive periodontitis in adjunctive to Augmentin
- Moreover, periodontal abscess

SIDE EFFECTS:

Oral: Bitter and/or metallic taste, oral candidosis

GI: Nausea, vomiting, epigastric distress and abdominal distress

CNS: Dizziness, vertigo, headache paraesthesia and numbness (sensory neuropathies)

Interaction with alcohol: It produces disulfiram-like reaction in alcoholic patients, (manifestations include flushing, tachycardia, hyperventilation, panic and distress). [2]

Availability:

Oral: 250, 500 mg tablet. [3]
Parenteral: 500 mg for injection

Dosage:

Dose of 250 mg t.i.d or 500 mg t.i.d for 7 days is use.

TINIDAZOLE:

It is a second-generation nitroimidazole.
Its antimicrobial spectrum is similar to that of metronidazole.
It is use as an alternative to metronidazole.
It differs from metronidazole in that it has shorter course of treatment.

Its **uses** include:

- Amebiasis
- Giardiasis
- Amoebic liver abscess

DILOXANIDE:

Diloxanide Furoate, is available and used usually after the treatment with metronidazole. When the Amebiasis has subsided and patient becomes asymptomatic.

Side effects are minimal and may include GI disturbances. However, it has highest safety profile. [1]

DENTAL CONSIDERATION:

- Determine the reason for taking these drugs.
- These drugs may predispose patient to dry mouth leading to increased susceptibility for dental caries, periodontal diseases and candidiasis.
- Ask the patient not to consume alcohol because of 'disulfiram-like reaction' may occur especially with metronidazole.
- Avoid use of alcohol containing mouth rinses (e-g Listerine).
- Oral candidosis may occur with the use of metronidazole; therefore, the dentist should address it. Topical use of anti-fungal drugs is helpful in eliminating the lesion. (For detail, see chapter 34 Anti-fungal drugs).
- Advocate fluoride home treatment.
- Dry mouth may be treated with sugar free chewing gum (Xylitol), tart and frequent sip of water during mealtime. [10]

FUNGAL INFECTION

Fungi are non-motile eukaryotic cells. Approximately 50 species are found to be pathogenic to humans. Infection caused by these fungi is known as Mycoses, which are generally associated with skin and mucous membrane. For the last few decades the prevalence of serious systemic fungal infection has been increased because of many factors, of which most important are the use of broad spectrum antibiotics (as an empirical therapies, which destroys many normal flora of human bodies) and the use of immunosuppressive drugs or cancer chemotherapies as well as patients infected with HIV (AIDS). All these factors contributed to the increased incidence of disseminated infections.

Fungal infections are of two types:

1. *Superficial fungal infection includes dermatomycoses and candidiasis (oral, vaginal thrush and the skin infection).*
2. *Disseminated or systemic fungal disease includes Candidiasis, Cryptococcal meningitis, pulmonary Aspergillosis and Endocardidtis.*

Fungi classification:
Clinically it has been classified into four main types;

1. *Yeast (Cryptococcus neoformans)*
2. *Yeast-like fungi that makes a structure similar to mycelium (Candida albicans)*
3. *Filamentous fungi having true mycelium (Aspergillus)*
4. *Either dimorphic fungi, that may grow as yeasts or filamentous fungi depending upon the type of nutrients. (Histoplasma Capsulatum).* [1]

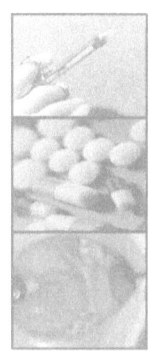

CHAPTER 34

Anti-Fungal Drugs

CLASSIFICATION:

Naturally occurring antibiotics:

Polyenes:
Amphotericin B
Nystatin

Echinocandins:
Anidulafungin
Caspofungin

Synthetic antibiotics:

Azoles:
Fluconazole
Miconazole
Ketoconazole
Clotrimazole
Econazole
Sulconazole
Posaconazole
Voriconazole

Other antibiotics:

Flucytosine

Terbinafine [1]

MODE OF ACTION:

Amphotericin B belongs to polyene group, which has an effect on cell membrane of fungi. It produces pore in the cell membrane forming an ion channel for the transport of ions. This leads to gross disturbance of ions including loss of potassium ions from inside the cells. Amphotericin binds avidly to the ergosterol of cell membrane of fungi; it has less affinity for the cell membrane of mammals and no ability to bind at all with bacterial cell wall. Therefore, it is highly specific on fungi that are advantageous in the sense that it causes less harm to humans.

Echinocandins, inhibit the synthesis of glucose polymer, 1,3-beta-glucan, which is important for maintaining the integrity of fungal cell wall. If this glucose polymer is not present, the fungal cell wall will lyse and ultimately breakdown of cell will occur.

Azoles, act by inhibiting the cytochrome P450 3A enzyme of fungi, which converts lanosterol to ergosterol (the main sterol of fungal cell membrane). As a result, the ergosterol will diminish leading to alteration in fluidity of the cell membrane. Ultimate action is the inhibition of replication process. [1]

INDICATIONS:

Dental uses: [6,7]

a) For pseudomembranous candidosis (thrush)
    Amphotericin or Nystatin Lozenges are use.
    If persist after the use of above lozenges then patient may be suspicious of HIV positive, then use of Fluconazole and Itraconazole can be helpful.

b) For angular stomatitis/cheilitis
Topical application of Nystatin is very useful. It is sometimes associated with Staphylococcus aureus infection so concomitant use of fusidic acid cream at the corner of mouth is also curative.

c) Denture-induced stomatitis
This is an erythematous condition of mucosa of hard palate underlying the denture, usually found in smokers.
Treatment includes, removal of the denture plus topical use of Nystatin or Amphotericin until erythema resolves.
Candida albicans from denture can be removed by washing it with 0.1% hypochlorite solution or diluted 0.12% Chlorhexidine.

d) Chronic hyperplastic candidosis (candidal Leukoplakia)
Nystatin 100,000 Units q.i.d for 7-10 days
Amphotericin 10 mg for 7-10 days
Fluconazole 50mg/day for 7-14 days
(Note: Continue antifungal therapy even 2 weeks following disappearance of signs and symptoms).

See also section on Individual Drugs below.

SIDE EFFECTS:

They decrease the effect of Cytochrome p450 enzyme system therefore, when use concomitantly with other drugs (like Warfarin), dose of Warfarin should be increase.

See also section on Individual Drugs below.

INDIVIDUAL DRUGS:

1). Amphotericin B:

Route of administration, as it is poorly absorbed from GIT. Therefore, for systemic infection it is given intravenously mixed with other lipid preparations or liposomes. In addition, for skin or mucus membrane lesions it is given topically. Only for upper GI track infection, it is given per oral.

Indications:

It is use mainly for systemic infection via intravenous administration. (Candidiasis and Aspergillosis)
In addition, use for Cryptococcal meningitis as it penetrates into inflamed tissue very well (though donot cross the blood-brain barrier when no inflammation is present).

Side effects:

- Renal toxicity is the most common side effect.
- Fever and chills may occur due to repeated intravenous administration (premedication with Corticosteroids or anti-pyretic may prevent this condition).
- Hypokalemia may occur in 25% of patients.
- Neurotoxicity can produce following intrathecal injection.
- Skin rashes can result following topical application.
- Thrombophlebitis occurs following intravenous injection (this can be prevented by adding heparin to the infusion).
- Hypomagnesaemia may produce leading to anaemia.

Availability:

Topical 3% cream, lotion and ointment
Parenteral 50mg per vial solution

2). Nystatin:

Route of administration, as it has systemic toxicity so; it is only applied topically or as an oral agent (swish and swallow or swish and spit).

Indications:

Oral candidiasis (thrush)

Side effects:

This may include *nausea and vomiting* but they are rare.

It decreases the effect of Cytochrome p450 enzyme system therefore, when use concomitantly with other drugs (like Warfarin), dose of warfarin should be increase.

Availability:

Topical 100,000 units /gram cream, ointment, powder.

Oral 500,000 unit tablets

3). Echinocandins:

This includes *Anidulafungin* and *Caspofungin*.

Route of administration: If GI absorption is poor, it is also given intravenously.

Indications:

It includes systemic infections like Candidiasis and Aspergillosis (that are refractory to Amphotericin)

Side effects:

They cause histamine-mediated side effects like

- Fever
- Rashes and phlebitis.

4). Fluconazole:

Route of Administration: As it is well absorbed from GIT so it can be given per oral.

It is also given parenterally (intravenously).

Indications:

Use for *fungal meningitis* as its concentration reaches to CSF.

Also used for *Oral fungal infection* because its concentration also reaches to saliva.

Its concentration also reaches to vaginal secretion, skin and nails therefore, use for fungal infection of vagina, skin and nails.

Side effects:

Stevens-Johnson syndrome has been reported especially in patients with HIV.

Other rare side effects include; Nausea, Headache, Abdominal pain

Hepatitis

Availability:

Oral 50,100, 150, 200 mg tablets

Parenteral 2 mg/ml in 200 and 400 ml vials.

5). Miconazole:

Route of Administration: It is applied topically.

Indications:

Use mainly for Oral candidiasis.

Use for GI fungal infections.

Side effects:

GI disturbances

Blood Dyscrasias (symptoms include fever, poor wound healing, bleeding).

Pruritis.

It is contraindicated to the patient with hepatic impairment.

Availability:

Topical 2% cream, powder, spray.

Parenteral 10 mg/ml for injection.

6). Flucytosine:

Routes of Administration: It is mostly given intravenously but can also be given orally.

Indications:

It is combined with Amphotericin B for synergistic effect.

Uses for systemic infections include:

Candidiasis

Cryptococcal meningitis (as it is widely distributed throughout the body including CSF)

Side effects:

- GI disturbances
- Anaemia
- Neutropenia
- Thrombocytopenia
- Hair loss (alopecia) [1]

Availability:

Oral 250, 500 mg capsules

DENTAL CONSIDERATION:

- Determine the need for using anti-fungal drugs.
- Report any signs or symptoms associated with allergic reaction like fever, skin rashes and anaphylaxis.
- If patient shows signs of blood dyscrasias as mostly associated with miconazole refer patient to primary care physician. (Manifestation of blood dyscrasias include fever, bleeding and poor wound healing). [10]
- Manage oral candidal infection with appropriate antibiotic usage and proper management according to individual infection.
- Prescribe topical anti-fungal agents for specific diseases. For more detail, see section on Dental use of anti-fungal drugs.

VIRUSES

Viruses are small infective agents that cannot reproduce outside their host cells. They are 20-30 nm in size. When they are outside their host (free-living), they are known as virions.

Composition, include DNA or RNA (segments of nucleic acid) which is surrounded by protein coat known as capsid. Together these two are known as nucleocapsid.

Some viruses also acquire lipoprotein coat from their host, which they derive from their host-infected cell membrane.

Virus Function:

As we know viruses cannot replicate outside their host therefore they need their host metabolic machinery to replicate. So the coat portion of virus binds to receptor in human body (receptor may be hormones, neurotransmitters, ion channels, integral membrane glycoproteins, etc.)

After binding the receptor-virus complex enters into the cell (by receptor-mediated endocytosis). Inside the cell, viruses then use the host metabolic machinery to synthesize their nucleic acids and proteins in order to make new virus particles.

Host response to virus:

Host response to virus is defensive in nature. The first barrier that a virus encounters while entering into the human host is skin, from which the virus cannot evade through. However, the virus can gain access into the body via breached skin and mucous membrane. As virus gain access to human host, a cluster of T-cell lymphocytes is deployed to recognize foreign antigen. This foreign antigen when infect a normal cell, that particular cell present on its surface a receptor known as MHC 1 molecule.

This MHC 1 molecule is target by T-cell lymphocytes and at the same time many lytic enzymes are released form infected cells (e-g perforins).[1]

Viruses are broadly classified into two categories based on their type of nucleic acids.

So, the Pathogenic viruses to human beings include:

DNA viruses

Herpes viruses (cause chicken pox, shingles, cold sores, glandular fever)

Poxviruses (cause small pox)

Adenoviruses (cause sore throat and conjunctivitis)

Human Papilloma viruses (cause warts)

RNA viruses

Paramoxyviruses (cause measles, mumps and respiratory track infections).

Picarnoviruses (cause colds, meningitis and poliomyelitis).

Retroviruses (cause acquired immuno-deficiency syndrome).

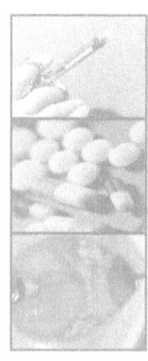

CHAPTER 35

Antiviral Drugs

CLASSIFICATION:

Viral DNA polymerase inhibitors

For CMV:
Aciclovir
Famciclovir
Penciclovir
Valaciclovir

For Herpes virus:
Ganciclovir
Valganciclovir
Foscarnet
Cidafovir

Nucleoside reverse trasciptase inhibitors

For Hepatitis B:
Adefovir
Entecavir
Lamivudine

For HIV:

Abacavir

Didanosine

Emtricitabne

Stavudine

Tenofovir

zidovudine

lamivudine

Biopharmaceuticals and immunomodulators

For Hepatitis B and C:

Interferon-alpha

For Respiratory virus:

Ribavirin

Palvizumab

For Herpes virus:

Inosine Prabonex [2]

MODE OF ACTIONS:

DNA polymerase inhibitors: Herpes virus-encoded enzyme phosphorylates acyclovir to monophosphate. Then the host cell kinases convert this monophosphate into triphosphate. This acyclovir triphosphate competes with deoxyguanosine triphosphate for viral DNA polymerase causing premature DNA chain termination. They are less effective against Host cell enzymes.

Nucleoside reverse transciptase inhibitors: Host cell enzymes, to give the 5′ triphosphate derivative, phosphorylate them. This competes with the equivalent host cellular triphosphate substrates for DNA synthesis by viral reverse transcriptase. As a result, this 5-triphosphate incorporates into the growing DNA chain resulting in chain termination.

Biopharmaceutical and immunomodulators: They are agents, which get recruit against virus infections.

Interferons are synthesize by mammalian cells as well as commercially prepared by recombinant DNA technology. Interferon Gamma is mainly produced by T-cell lymphocytes in response to both viral and non-viral antigens (like bacteria and their products, fungi etc). T and B-lymphocytes, macrophages and fibroblasts in response to viruses and cytokines produce interferon beta.

Interferon induces an enzyme in the host cell ribosome that halts the translation of viral mRNA into viral protein thus inhibiting viral replication.

Inosine prabonex: is an immunomodulators (those agent which moderate immune response according to the action of viruses). It is thought to have an interference with the nucleic acid synthesis.

INDICATIONS:

1. Cidofovir and Foscarnet are use for CMV (cytomegalo virus infections).
2. Aciclovir, famciclovir, valaciclovir and insosine prabonex are use for herpes viruses infections (chicken pox, shingles, genital herpes, mucocutaneous herpes and herpes encephalitis),
3. Use as a prophylaxis for patient who is jeopardized for herpes virus infection (e-g patient with latent virus in trigeminal nerve ganglion). Such patient can develop post-herpetic neuralgia.
4. Use as a prophylaxis for patient who is to be treated with radiotherapy or immuno-suppressant drugs.
5. Use as a prophylaxis for patient with recurrent genital herpes infections.
6. Zidovudine, Abacavir and Saquinavir is use for HIV infection. (Often use in combination with reverse tranciptase inhibitors).
7. Treatment for HIV may include;

- Monitor plasma viral concentration and CD_4 cell count.
- Use combination regimen of at least 3 drugs (e-g one from protease inhibitor and 2 from reverse transcriptase inhibitors).
- Start treatment before immuno deficiency become evident.
- Make the plasma viral concentration less as much as possible.
- If plasma viral concentration is increasing then change the treatment regimen to another group of drugs.

Dental uses:

- Use for herpetic stomatitis caused by HSV (herpes simplex virus).
- Use for recurrent herpes labialis (cold sore).
- Use for herpes zoster (shingles) caused by VZV (Varicella-Zoster virus). Which usually targets oral mucosa especially fauces and soft palate [4,7]

SIDE EFFECTS:

DNA polymerase inhibitors:
GI disturbances
Dermatological problems
Nephrotoxicity
Blood disorders
Ocular problems

Nucleoside reverse transcriptase inhibitors:
GI disturbances
Blood disorders
Dermatological effects

Pancreatitis

Liver damage

Lipodystrophy

Lactic acidosis

Biopharmaceuticals and immuno modulators:

GI disturbances including anorexia

Flu-like effect

Fever

Fatigue

Hyperuricaemia

INDIVIDUAL DRUGS:

1. **Valacyclovir:**

   In case of herpetic stomatitis, it is given in 500 mg dose, b.i.d for 5 days.

   In case of shingles, it is also given in 1 g dose t.i.d for 7 days.

   It is available in cream form, applied topically on cold sore.

2. **Acyclovir:**

   In case of Chicken pox, it is given in a dose of 800 mg, 5 times a day for 7 days. [7]

DENTAL CONSIDERATION:

- Document the need for therapy of anti-viral drugs.
- Take history about the type and onset of symptoms.
- Treat all patients as infective.
- Take precautions for infections, like wearing of glasses (for prevention of cornea), wearing of double gloves (reduce the chances of infection by six times), surgical cap and gown in a fully sterilized form.

- Some viral infections having oral manifestations that should be treated by dentist, by using topical anti-viral drugs and related managment.
- Oral manifestations of viral infections include vesicles formation, rupturing of vesicles into clusters, burning sensation, gingivostomatitis and cold sore formation. [6]
- Commonly used topical drugs are acyclovir and valacyclovir. For further detail, see chapter 38, section on viral infections.

LOCAL ANAESTHETICS

Definition:

Local anaesthetic is an agent whose anaesthetic action is limited to an area of the body determined by the state of its application; it produces its effect by blocking nerve conduction.

While **topical anaesthetic** is a local anaesthetic applied directly to the area to be anesthetized, usually the mucous membrane and the skin.

(Ref: Dorland's Medical Dictionary)

Ideal properties of Local anaesthetics:

- They should be non-irritating to the tissue to which they are applied.
- They should cause no permanent alteration to the nerve structure.
- They should have low systemic toxicity.
- The duration of action should be long enough to permit completion of dental procedure yet not too long to require an extended recovery.
- The time of onset should be as short as possible.
- They should be effective regardless of administration, whether injected or applied topically to the soft tissues (mucous membrane of mouth).[5]

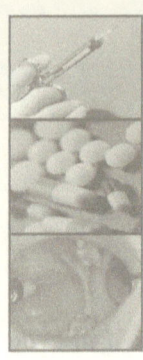

CHAPTER 36

Local Anaesthetics

Local anaesthetics are those agents, which produce loss of sensation in localized area of body caused by depression of excitation in nerve endings or by inhibition of nerve conduction in peripheral nerves.

CLASSIFICATION:

Esters:
Cocaine
Procaine
Propoxycaine
Tetracaine
Benzocaine
Dyclonine

Amides:
Lidocaine
Etidocaine
Mepivacaine
Bupivacaine
Articaine
Prilocaine

MECHANISM OF ACTION:

Electrophysiology of nerve conduction:

A nerve possesses resting membrane potential of—70 mV. The interior of nerve is more negative relative to the exterior.

Step 1: when a stimulus (like chemical, mechanical, thermal or electrical) excites the nerve an initial phase of *slow depolarization* occurs the interior electrical potential becomes slightly less negative (that is the Na$^+$ ions move from outside to the inside). When this falling potential reaches a critical level, known as *threshold level or firing threshold*, an extremely *rapid phase of depolarization* results that is the abundance of Na$^+$ ions move from outside to the inside). This rapid phase of depolarization in turn results in reversal of electrical potential (that is exterior is more negative than interior).An electrical potential of +40 mV is now created at the interior.

Step 2: After depolarization, a *phase of repolarization* occurs. In which the K$^+$ *ions* move rapidly from inside to the outside resulting in again—60 to-90 mV potential.

These two steps require a time of one millisecond; step 1, (0.3 m Sec) and step 2 (0.7 m Sec).

Local anaesthetics interfere with the excitation of nerve in one of the following ways;

1. Altering the firing threshold (threshold level)
2. Altering the resting potential of nerve membrane
3. By decreasing the rate of depolarization
4. By increasing the rate of repolarisation

Local anaesthetics act on the nerve membrane. How it acts is represented by many theories, amongst which only two are widely accepted. We will discuss here only these two theories. [5]

1. Membrane expansion theory:

This theory is for a local anaesthetic agent, which is lipid-soluble (e-g Benzocaine) this agent does not possess cationic feature.

This theory states that local anaesthetic, which is a lipid soluble substance penetrates into the hydrophobic region of nerve membrane, here it alters the configuration of nerve membrane (lipoprotein matrix) in such a way that this agent causes an expansion of nerve membrane so that the ion-gated sodium channel gets partially or completely blocked. Hence, the excitation as well as conduction of membrane potential is halted. However, it is still not completely evident that membrane potential is entirely blocked by this membrane expansion per se.

2. Specific receptor theory:

This theory states that the local anaesthetic binds with the specific receptors on the sodium channel. These receptors are present on the sodium channel either on the outer-side or on the interior axoplasmic side. As the local anaesthetic gain access to these receptors the Na^+ ions permeability is decreased and hence conductance is hampered. [5]

Working of Local anaesthetics:

Calcium ions are mainly responsible for the conduction of sodium ions channels in the nerve cells. Calcium ions are bound to channel receptor's site in the cell membrane when they become unbound the conduction of sodium permeability in the nerve membrane increases.

- First, the calcium ions get unbound from the cell membrane.
- That allows the local anaesthetics to bind with the receptor on sodium channels.
- That in turn produces blockade of the sodium channels.

- Decrease in sodium conductance in turns lead to slowing the rate of depolarization.
- That leads to the failure of achieving desirable threshold level.
- Therefore, there is lack of development of propagated action potential.
- That ultimately led to the blockage of Conduction.

Biotransformation:

Ester Local Anaesthetics:

They are hydrolyze in the plasma by an enzyme known as pseudocholinesterase. Because of hydrolysis, new products are formed known as PABA (in case of procaine) and diethylamine alcohol. PABA is excreted unchanged in the urine whereas diethylamine alcohol undergoes further metabolism before excretion.

Allergic reaction that occurs, from esters LA is in response to PABA not the primary compound procaine.

The rate of hydrolysis of different esters is related to its potential toxicity. For example, rate of hydrolysis of tetracaine is the lowest (that is 0.3 μmol/ml/hr) so its toxicity is highest.

Whereas the rate of hydrolysis of chloprociane is the highest (that is 4.7 μmol /ml/hr) so its toxicity is lowest.

Amide Local Anaesthetics:

They are metabolized mainly in the liver; however, Prilocaine is metabolized in the lungs in addition to liver.

Hence, hepatic perfusion plays an important role in the biotransformation of amide LA. Conditions like *cardiac failure, hypotension and poor liver function (cirrhosis)* make the rate of hydrolysis of this amide LA very slow thus adding to the potential systemic toxicity of LA.

The biotransformation product of *Prilocaine* is *orthotoluidine*, responsible for methamoglobinemia. Signs and symptoms include respiratory distress, lethargy, cyanotic mucous membrane and nail beds, chocolate brown venous blood. The diagnosis is made when cyanotic condition remains unresponsive to the administration of oxygen.

The metabolic products of *Lidocaine* are *glycinexylidide and monoethylglycinexylidide* which are thought to be responsible for sedative effect.

Action of local anaesthetics:

The systemic effect of local anaesthetic is related to its blood or plasma level.

As local anaesthetics are chemicals that reversibly, block the action potential in all excitable nerve membranes. They have the following systemic effects.

On CNS:

Anti-convulsing effect:
This effect occurs at very low blood level (that is at 0.5-4 µgram / ml).

This level is achieve at a dose of 2-3 mg/kg given intravenously at the rate of 40-50 mg /minute.

Mechanism: As epileptic patient demonstrate very high excitable levels of conduction in the brain region (epileptic focus) so, local anaesthetics raise the threshold level by decreasing the excitation of these neurons.

This constitutes the therapeutic level for local anaesthetic drugs.
Pre-convulsive state:
When local anaesthetic level increases from that of therapeutic level (that's blood level reaches upto 4.5 to 7 µgram /ml) *preconvulsive signs and symptoms appear.*

These include shivering, generalized light-headedness, slurred speech, dizziness, visual disturbances, auditory disturbances, muscle twitching, tremors of muscles of face and distal extremities, numbness of tongue and circumoral region, warmth and flushing of skin and disorientation.

Convulsion state:

This occurs at a blood level above 7.5 µgram /ml.

Mechanism:

As we know that in cerebral cortex there are pathways known as inhibitory and facilitatory (excitatory) pathways.

In normal condition, there is a balance between inhibitory and facilitatory impulses in the CNS (cerebral cortex).

At preconvulsive stage, the inhibitory impulse is more depressed than the facilitatory impulse.

At convulsion stage, the inhibitory impulse is very depressed whereas the facilitatory impulse gets dominate.

At further stage both inhibitory and facilitatory impulses are inhibited leading to total CNS depression.

Analgesia:

Another action of local anaesthetic on CNS is analgesia, which is produce by increasing pain threshold in CNS.

ON CVS:

Local anaesthetics decrease the electrical excitability of myocardium as they decrease the electrical excitability of peripheral neurons.

Therefore, they decrease the rate of conduction and force of contraction of myocardium.

The therapeutic blood level of Lidocaine is 1.8-6 µgram/ml, which makes lidocaine used as an anti-arrhythmic drug.

The dose for anti-arrhythmic effect is 1-1.5 mg/kg body weight, given intravenously at the rate of 25-50 mg/min.

Over Dose:

It occurs at blood level above 6 µg/ml, the signs and symptoms include talkativeness, apprehension, excitability, muscular twitching, tremor on facial muscles and distal extremities, dysarthria, euphoria, failure to follow commands, metallic taste, visual and auditory disturbances, drowsiness, loss of consciousness and elevated blood pressure, heart rate and respiratory rate.

Moderte to high overdose:

Signs and symptoms include depressed blood pressure, heart rate and respiratory rate.

On peripheral vasculature:

On blood vessels the action of local anaesthetic is vasodilation (except Cocaine which causes vasoconstriction) leading to hypotension.

At approaching overdose, level (4-5 µg/ml) there is mild degree of hypotension due to relaxation of vascular smooth muscles.

At moderate overdose level (> 6 µg /ml) there is profound hypotension with decreased myocardial contractility, cardiac output and peripheral resistance.

At lethal overdose level (approx. 10 µg/ml), there is a massive vasodilation and decreased myocardial contractility and heart rate (sinus bradycardia and CVS collapse).

Bupivacaine is known to be cardiotoxic as it may potentiate severe fatal ventricular fibrillation.

On Respiratory system:

At low doses, they produce relaxation of bronchial smooth muscles.

At higher doses, they produce *respiratory arrest* due to *Generalized CNS depression.*

On Local tissue:

Locally they act on skeletal muscles like medial and lateral pterygoid muscles or other muscles of facial expression when given intra-orally.

They temporarily damage the skeletal muscles and irritate them. Then muscle regeneration occurs within 2 weeks of local anaesthetic administration. [5]

INDICATIONS:

- Use for local infiltration. (In which small terminal nerve endings are flooded with solution of local anaesthetic)
- Use for field block. (In which local anaesthetic solution is deposited near the larger terminal nerve branches)
- Use for regional nerve block. (In which local anaesthetic solution is deposited at a site away from the site of operation) Example in dentistry include inferior alveolar nerve block, other examples include branchial plexus and intercostal nerve blocks.
- Use for surface anaesthesia. (In which local anaesthesia is either topically applied or sprayed on mucus membrane of oral cavity and nose)
- Use for intravenous regional anaesthesia. (In which local anaesthetic is given IV distal to the pressure cuff to arrest blood flow, it remains effective until reperfusion of blood).
- Use for Spinal anaesthesia. (In which Local anaesthetic is deposited in to subarachnoid space possessing CSF, to act on spinal root and spinal cor). Examples include abdominal, pelvis or leg surgery.
- Use for epidural anaesthesia. (In which local anaesthetic is deposited into the epidural space) example includes painless delivery of childbirth.

- Use for dysarrhythmia, the local anaesthetic is given intravenously to the patient within therapeutic dose level.
- Use for epilepsy, the local anaesthetic (particularly Lidocaine) is use in therapeutic doses to treat epilepsy.
- Use for haemorrhage control, those local anaesthetics, which contain epinephrine in concentration of 1:50,000 are use to control bleeding at the site of operation.
- Use for neuropathic pain, for example trigeminal neuralgia. In which LA is given as an infiltration at the site of pain.

SIDE EFFECTS:

Systemic side effects:

At blood levels 7.5-10 µg /ml

CNS: confusion, agitation, tremors progressing to convulsions and respiratory depression

At blood levels 5-10 µg /ml

CVS: Myocardial depression, vasodilation (severe hypotension), ECG alteration

At blood levels 10 µg /ml or above

Massive peripheral vasodilation, intensive myocardial depression and cardiac arrest occur.

Allergic reaction: may occur in response to LA but this has decreased due to the introduction of amide local anaesthetics.

Manifestations of allergic reactions are:

Skin (rashes, hives, itching and oedema)

GIT (nausea, vomiting, cramping and diarrhoea)

Respiratory system (wheezing and laryngeal oedema)

Exocrine glands (watery eyes and runny nose)

Genitourinary system (faecal and urinary incontinence)

Cardiovascular system (angioedema, hypotension)

At the end, Anaphylactic shock may occur but this severe condition is very rare.

Local side effects:

- Persistent anaesthesia or paraesthesia
- Soft-tissue injury may occur as the regional area is anaesthetized leading to numbness due to which a child patient may bite on his or her lip.
- Haematoma may form in cases where the needle is injected into the blood vessel while giving infiltration or field block.
- Pain on injection can be experienced while giving local anaesthetic injection, which is due to the barbed needle after hitting the bone.
- Burning sensation is felt because of the acidic pH of LA solution.
- Sloughing of tissues can occur, for example in case of epithelial desquamation due to prolong use of topical anaesthesia for more than 2 minutes.
- Sterile Abscess usually occurs on hard palate mucosa due to injection of LA with epinephrine. Epinephrine produces prolong ischemia of the soft tissues. [5]

INDIVIDUAL DRUGS:

Preparations available:

1. **Lidocaine:**
   Xylocaine, 2% Lidocaine (20 mg/ml), with epinephrine 1:100,000
   Lignospan forte, 2% Lidocaine HCL with epinephrine 1:50,000
   Lignospan standard, 2% Lidocaine HCL with epinephrine 1:100,000

2. **Mepivacaine:**
   Scandonest 3% plain, contains 3% Mepivacaine HCL

Scandonest 2%L, contains 2% Mepivacaine HCL with Levonordefrin in 1:20,000 concentration

Carbocaine 3%, contains 3% Mepivacaine without vasoconstrictor

3. **Prilocaine:**

   4% Citanest plain, contains 4% prilocaine without vasoconstrictor

   4% Citanest Forte, contains 4% prilocaine with epinephrine 1:200,000

4. **Articaine:**

   Septocaine, contains 4% Articaine HCL with epinephrine 1:100,000

5. **Bupivacaine:**

   Marcaine, contains 0.5% Bupivacaine with epinephrine 1:200,000

Topical Preparations:

1. **Lidocaine:**

   Lidocaine base, (Xylocaine) Aerosal 10 mg/metered spray

   Lidocaine HCL, (Xylocaine viscous) Oral topical solution 20 mg/ml

2. **Tetracaine:**

   (Supracaine) Aerosal 0.5 mg/metered spray

3. **EMLA:**

   Eutectic mixture of local anaesthetics which contains Lidocaine 2.5% and prilocaine 2.5% in a ratio 1:1 by weight.

   Availability:

   It is supplied in 5g or 30g tube or as an EMLA anaesthetic disc.

It is good for skin application however it is also used for oral mucous membrane as evident from number of experiments on patients in dental office.

It is given 1 hour before the start of procedure; the effective numbness of skin is achieved after 1 hour reaching maximum after 2-3 hours and then lasts for 1-2 hours after removal. [5]

DENTAL CONSIDERATION:

- Take full medical history from patient including allergy to LA and any bad past experience with dental procedure or use of local anaesthetic injection.
- Document these conditions in particular if patient have history of heart failure, Angina, MI, hypertension, thyroid crisis, epilepsy (seizures). Also note if patient have implanted heart valve, artificial pace maker, implanted cardioverter/ defibrillator and stent. [8]
- Forms of anaemia, methamoglobinemia represent *relative contraindication* to the administration of LA Prilocaine.
- After completion of medical and dental history, put the patient in semi-supine position or preferably in supine position in order to avoid syncope at the time of LA administration.
- In order to avoid anxiety converse with patient frequently [5, 8]
- Ensure pain free LA injection administration, by applying antiseptic to mucous membrane followed by topical application of LA.
- Insert the needle gently into the mucous membrane and deposit local anaesthetic solution slowly at the rate of 1 ml/ minute.
- After depositing LA solution withdraw the needle gently and wait for LA to be effective (on average 4-5 minutes are required for all local anaesthetics to be effective). [5]

PART III

Pharmacology in Dental practice

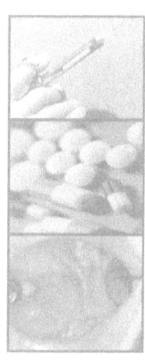

CHAPTER 37

Drugs for oral lesions

FUNGAL INFECTIONS

Fungal infection in oral mucosa is mainly caused by Candida species. Candida albicans is the main organism. In addition to C.albican, C.glabrata, C.tropicalis, C.krusei and C.parapsilosis are also involved.

Candida is commensal organism in the mouth so they are opportunistic, whenever they find an opportunity to cause infection. Some local and systemic factors will predispose oral cavity to the candidal infection.

The predisposing factors are:

Local: Tobacco smoking, mucosal ulceration, Denture wearing, Xerostomia, use of broad-spectrum antibiotics and local use of corticosteroid and immunosuppressive drugs

Systemic: Diabetes mellitus, iron-deficiency anaemia, acute leukaemia, malignant diseases, HIV infections and other immuno deficiency states

Pseudomembranous candidosis:

Clinical Features:

Thick white coating like milk curd on oral mucosa, (this can be wiped away leaving red, raw and bleeding base).

Treatment:

Topical use of Nystatin (Nilstat) is 100,000-unit q.i.d for 7-10 days.

Clotrimazole lozenge 10 mg chewable is also helpful.

If patient is HIV-infected, then Fluconazole 50 mg tablets per day for 10-14 days are useful.In addition to use of local anti fungal drugs, local factors should be removed, and systemic factors should be managed.

Angular Cheilitis:

Clinical features:

It is an infection present at the corner of mouth caused by either fungi or S.aureus or streptococci or both fungal and bacterial infection. It is usually present in elderly edentulous patients whose all teeth are extracted, they have low vertical dimension due to which furrows are formed at the corners of mouth, which are frequently contaminated with the drooling of saliva hence, providing better habitat for infectious microorganisms.

Treatment:

Apply miconazole gel 24 mg/ml at the corners of the mouth.

Caution: Avoid in pregnancy, it can potentiate Warfarin anticoagulation effect but not at these small doses. [6, 7]

VIRAL INFECTIONS

Main viral infections that can present in Oral cavity include:
HSV Type 1 and 2 = (herpetic stomatitis)
VZV = (chicken pox and shingles) [Herpes Zoster]

Herpetic stomatitis:

Clinical Features:

An incubation period is about 5 days; prodromal symptoms fever and malaise appear followed by numerous small vesicles in the oral cavity after 1 or 2 day of prodromal symptoms. The mouth becomes extremely uncomfortable and become associated with gingivostomatitis.

The vesicle soon ulcerate and become secondarily infected which is associated with regional lymphadenitis.

Treatment:

Treatment is oral valacyclovir 500 mg b.i.d for 5 days. Alternatively, Acyclovir (do mouth rinse and swallow) 200-400 mg per day for 7 days.

Herpes Labialis: (Cold sore)

(After the primary infection, latent virus can become activated and may cause cold sore)

Clinical Features:

It includes prodromal symptoms such as burning sensation and paraesthesia then after one hour or two, vesicles form at the mucocutaneous junction of the lips.

Treatment:

Treatment includes acyclovir Cream applied topically on the site of lesion. Alternatively, pencilcovir applied 2-hourly is more potent.

Treatment should be started as soon as burning sensation or paraesthesia is felt.

Herpetic whitlow:

Clinical Features:

It is a primary infection on non-oral site (that's finger usually index finger) that occurs because of contact with infected saliva or vesicle fluid.

Treatment:

It includes topical use of acyclovir on affected site; in addition, attendant should wear gloves while applying cream on the infected vesicles in order to avoid contact with it.

Herpes Zoster of Trigeminal area:

Clinical features:

In this, painful vesicles are formed at the site of trigeminal dermatome areas. Regional lymph nodes are enlarged and tender. The vesicles then crust and heal after about one week.

Treatment:

In treatment, oral acyclovir 800 mg five times a day is given for 7 days. In addition analgesics (e-g ibuprofen 400 mg t.i.d or Diclofenac 50 mg) or steroids (e-g prednisolone) may be given to relief acute phase of pain.

BACTERIAL INFECTIONS

Primary Syphilis:

Clinical features:

Primary chancre usually occurs 3-4 weeks after infection, the nodule breaks down and forms round ulcer with raised everted and indurate edges.Lesions occur at the site of lip, tip of tongue or rarely other oral sites.

Secondary syphilis:

Clinical features:

This phase occurs 1-4 months after an infection. It is characterized by fever, malaise, headache and sore throat, generalized lymphodenopathy and stomatitis.Oral lesions contain ulcers which is covered by greyish membrane (appear like snail's track ulcer) or coalesce to form round mucous patches.

Tertiary syphilis:

Clinical features:

This phase occurs about 3 or more years after an infection.

Salient feature is *gumma* formation, which begins with swelling that undergoes necrosis and form deep indolent ulcer. It then heals with scarring and may distort the palate or tongue or it may perforate the hard palate or may destroy the uvula. *Leukoplakia* is another feature in tertiary syphilis stage.

Treatment:

Penicillin is the drug of choice. However, erythromycin and tetracycline has also been effective. A specialist should do treatment.

RECURRENT APHTHOUS STOMATITIS

Minor Aphthae:

Clinical Features:
They include ulcers that are shallow, rounded, and 5-7 mm in diameter. They are most the common type, present on non-keratinized mucosa (lining mucosa). They heal without scarring and within 10 days. They recur at 1-4 months interval.

Major Aphthae:

Clinical features:
They include ulcers that are about 1-3 cm in diameter. They may occur any where in the oral cavity including keratinized mucosa (masticatory mucosa). Common sites are oro-pharynx, tonsillar pillar areas, soft palate and lips.

Herpetiform Aphthae:

Clinical features:
They are 1-2 mm in diameter. They are present in hundreds or dozens, which may also coalesce to form large ulcers. They are associated with severe discomfort.

Treatment:
For all aphthous ulcers, Hydrocortisone hemisuccinate (Corlan) 2.5 mg pellets are chewed to dissolve in mouth three times a day for 2 months. For acute relief of pain so that patient can eat comfortably, take a mixture *of* equal amount of *Diphenhydramine (Benadryl) and milk of magnesia* and do mouth rinse for 30 seconds before taking meal. Triamcinolone dental paste is also helpful in forming protective layer over the ulcers thus decreasing its discomfort.

Alternatively, capsules of tetracycline 250 mg is stir in water and held in mouth for 2-3 minutes three times a day. In addition, mouth rinse 0.2% Chlorhexidine is held in mouth for one-minute at least three times a day. It has claimed to reduce the discomfort of ulcers.

LICHEN PLANUS

Clinical features:

Reticular type lichen planus is asymptomatic, bilaterally present and consists of interlacing white lines on the posterior region of buccal mucosa. They have an erythematous background, which may also found in association with candidiasis.

Erosive type lichen planus is often associated with pain and clinically manifest as atrophic, erosive and ulcerated lesion. White fine radiating striations are found bordering the lesions such borders are sensitive to heat, spicy food and acid.

Treatment:

In mild cases, 0.05% fluocinonide gel (Lidex 1.5 g tube) is applied to the affected areas after meal and at bedtime.

Nystatin (100,000 IU) oral Pastilles are used when fungal infection occurs with the use of corticosteroids.

In refractory cases, Tacrolimus 0.5% (protopic 15 g tube) is applied to the affected area b.i.d

VESICULOBULLOUS DISEASES

They present in the oral cavity in the form of an ulcer after the rupture of vesicle or bulla. *Vesicle* is a smaller blister containing clear fluid in it, while *bulla* is a larger vesicle greater than 5 mm in diameter.

Classification:

Intraepithelial vesiculobullous diseases:
Pemphigus vulgaris
Paraneoplastic pemphigus
Dariere's disease
Viral infection of oral mucosa (e-g HSV) (Also see "viral infections").

Subepithelial vesiculobullous diseases:
Erythema multiforme
Mucous membrane pemphigoid
Bullous lichen planus

Pemphigus vulgaris:

Clinical Features:
There is widespread bullous eruption on the skin and on oral mucosa. In some cases, the lesions are only limited to oral cavity. In oral-cavity, they frequently affect soft palate, buccal mucosa and lips. The bullous soon ruptures and form an irregular raged mucosal ulcers. It is also associated with desquamative gingivitis.

Treatment:
Primary treatment is with the use of corticosteroids prednisolone 80-100 mg per day.
Secondary treatment is with cyclophosphamide, cyclosporine and gold. In addition, Azathioprine 1-1.5 mg/kg O.D is also used.

Erythema multiforme:

Clinical features:
It has wide clinical features as the name indicates 'multiforme'.

It involves the skin and oral mucous membrane. In *Stevens Johnson* syndrome there is wide involvement of skin, oral cavity, genitilia and ocular mucosa (conjunctival scarring and visual disturbances).

Oral manifestations include, first erythematous patches, which become vesiculobullous blisters, the blister soon erodes as the bulla disintegrates. This forms an erosion of the lips accompanied by bleeding and crusting.

Skin manifestations are mostly present on hands and feet. They present as erythematous maculopapular rashes and vesiculobullous eruptions. They look like concentric rings (target lesions) in the centre of which lie intact or ruptured bulla.

Treatment:

In treatment, systemic corticosteroids use is controversial according to new research still they are the first choice of drugs.

Secondly, antibiotics are added to the regimen in order to prevent secondary infections. (For example Augmentin [amoxicillin plus clavulaunic acid] 625 mg t.i.d)

LUPUS ERYTHEMATOSUS

Clinical features:

Chronic cutaneous lupus erythematosus has lesions only on skin and oral mucous membrane.

Oral manifestations are lichen planus like plaques on palate and buccal mucosa. The lesions are localized and have numerous dilated blood vessels in a radial like arrangement coupled with whitish pinhead papules. On lips, the lesions are similar to those in mouth. The gingiva suffers from desquamative gingivitis.

Treatment:

Skin rashes are treated with topical steroids and sunscreen. If patient is resistant to topical therapy then systemic anti-malarial therapy is indicated. [6,7]

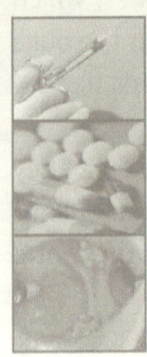

CHAPTER 38
Drugs for Oro-facial pain

BURNING MOUTH SYNDROME:

Clinical features:

It includes pain and aching sensation in whole mouth or part of it. This is also accompanied with dry mouth and altered taste sensation. Postmenopausal women are commonly affected; however, hormonal replacement therapy does not show any beneficial effect.

Treatment:

Treatment can be given in placebo, or with anticonvulsant drugs (lamotregine, topiramate) or antidepressant drugs (amitryptillin).

TRIGEMINAL NEURALGIA:

Clinical features:

It includes sharp, stabbing and electric shock like pain that occurs along the course of any branch of trigeminal nerve, ophthalmic, maxillary or mandibular division. It is of short duration, for few seconds to 1 min., triggered by just eating, washing face, or cold air of fan. Triggering areas are corner of mouth, cheeks, ala of nose and lateral brow. It mostly occurs in old age usually after 50 years that is commonly confused with odontalgia.

Treatment:

Treatment includes the use of anti convulsant drugs. For example Carbamazepine (tegral) 400-1200 mg per day, Gabapentin 600-3200 mg dose per day, Clonazepam (klonopin) 2-8 mg daily, Phenytoin (300-600) mg daily [7, 8]

MIGRAINE HEADACHE:

Clinical features:

It is a kind of headache that occurs on half side of face, splitting the head. *Prodromal signs* (from minutes to an hour), include visual aura, scotomata (retina), teichopsia (flashes) in case of classical migraine or circumoral and tongue tingling, vertigo, diplopia, transient visual disturbance, syncope, dysarthria in case of basilar migraine.

Headache starts with severe aching pain and patient prefers dark. It is initially localized then becoming generalized. After few hours migraine settles, followed by nausea and vomiting even during an attack. Deep sleep then ensues. *Scalp arteries are engorged* and pulsating during attack.

Treatment:

At the start of an attack,

- Paracetamol
- Serotonin receptor agonists, (side effects include coronary vasoconstriction and dysrhythmias)
- Sumatriptan
- Almotriptan

- Serotonin receptor partial agonist, (side effects include peripheral and coronary vessels vasoconstriction, contracts uterus and may damage the fetus)
- Ergotamine

As a prophylaxis, (prevention of an attack)

- Serotonin antagonist (side effects include weight gain and anti-muscarinic side effects)
- Pizotifen 0.5 mg at night
- Beta-blocker (side effects include bronchoconstriction)
- Propanolol 10-40 mg t.i.d
- Tricyclic anti-depressant
- Amitryptilin 10 mg at night [9]

TENSION HEADACHE:

Chronic benign tension headache is the most common of all headaches. It is usually associated with tension, anxiety, worries, following minor injuries and depression. Analgesic overuse is the prominent cause.

Clinical features:

It includes tight band sensation around head, pressure behind the eyes, throbbing and bursting sensation.

Treatment:

- Avoiding evident causes for example, bright lights.
- Physical treatments like massage, icepack and relaxation are very effective.
- Withdrawal of analgesics is another effective treatment.
- Use of antidepressants drugs if, indicated by patient's condition.

- Drugs for recurrent headache or migraine are also effective.

CLUSTER HEADACHE:

This unilateral headache lasts for several hours. It occurs in bouts of attacks. It occurs every night in bouts for one to two months. Then headache is subsided with the relief from attack.

Clinical features:
Main clinical feature is pain around the orbital region with nasal congestion.

Treatment:
Subcutaneous sumatriptan is the drug of choice.
Oxygen inhalational and verpamil, topiramate can be helpful.

EPISODIC PAROXYSMAL HEMICRANIA:

Clinical features:
A clinical feature is the same as cluster headache but duration is brief, less than 20 minutes.

Treatment:
It shows most effective response to indometacin.

SUNCT AND SUNA:

Sunct stands for, short lasting unilateral neuralgiform headache with conjunctival injection and tearing (5 seconds-2 minutes)
Suna stands for, short lasting unilateral neuralgiform headache with cranial autonomic symptoms

Treatment:
Immediate IV Lidocaine aborts an attack. [9]

GIANT CELL ARTERITIS:

Clinical features:

Headache and pain over the *inflamed temporal artery* occurs even, can occur with combing hair.

Pain on face, jaw and mouth occur due to inflammation of facial, maxillary and lingual branches of external carotid artery in GCA. Pain may worsen on eating, which is known as jaw claudication. It may or may not be associated with polymyalgia rheumatica PMR.

Treatment:

In GCA, the drug of choice is prednisone or methylprednisolone started in a dose of 40-60 mg per day in daily divided doses, which is then tapered off gradually. [9]

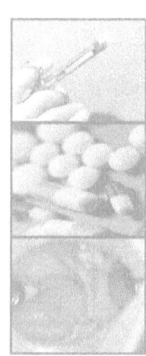

CHAPTER 39

Emergency Drugs in Dental office

ORAL DRUGS [8]

Nitroglycerin: (Nitrostat, Nitrolingual)

It belongs to a class of drug Nitrates, which is a potent vasodilator. For detail, see chapter 14 Nitrates.

Office Use:

When patient experiences chest pain and the dentist is suspicious of angina attack, while sitting on dental unit, Nitroglycerin 0.4 mg tablet is given sublingually in order to subside chest pain. If pain continues then Nitroglycerin can be given for the second and third time with an interval of 3-4 minutes.

Aspirin: (Disprin, Loprin)

When patient has an acute chest pain and it does not subside with Nitroglycerin then suspect acute MI attack. In this case, Aspirin

223

in a dose of 325 mg is given per oral. Four to five tablets of 75mg aspirin is given at a time.

In addition, Aspirin is also used when patient suffers an attack of stroke due to infarction. Stroke due to infarction must be differentiated from stroke due to haemorrhage, in stroke due to infarction the attack is all of a sudden and severe which later improves after some time, this is a diagnosis of infarction. While, in case of stroke due to haemorrhage patient condition deteriorates gradually this means, bleeding continues and haematoma is expanding. These are the clinical conditions that are diagnosed if; CT scan facility is not available. Hence, in case of stroke due to infarction we give aspirin in a dose of 300-600 mg orally.

Diphenhydramine: (Benadryl)

Chlorpheniramine: (Chlor-trimeton, Piriton)

When patient suffers mild allergic reaction (urticaria, pruritus and angioedema) in response to Local anaesthetic administration, immediately either Benadryl 50 mg or Chlor-trimeton 10 mg is given orally.

Prednisolone:

It is a corticosteroid given for an acute attack of asthma in a dose of 60 mg orally. In addition, Diphenhydramine or Chlorpheniramine (anti-histamines) are also given orally to subside an attack.

Sugar Candy or fruit juices:

They are kept for diabetic patients in case; the patient undergoes hypoglycaemia while sitting on dental chair.

PARENTERAL DRUGS [8]

Diphenhydramine: (Benadryl)

Chlorpheniramine: (Chlor-trimeton)

When patient suffers an allergic reaction bit severe than mild, such signs of erythema, pruritus and angioedema may occur then we can administer Benadryl 50mg or Chlor-trimeton 10 mg IM or IV.

Epinephrine:

It is also known as 'Life-saving Drug'. It is the only drug, which should be present in pre-loaded form all the time in dental office.

It is given in number of conditions like; when patient has severe allergic reaction such as respiratory difficulty (wheezing, dyspnoea and stridorous breathing). Then epinephrine is administered in a dose of 0.3 ml (1:1000) IM, IV or SC. When patient has an anaphylactic shock, (wheezing, stridor, cyanosis, nausea, vomiting, tachycardia, hypotension, cardiac arrest); Epinephrine is administered in a dose of 0.3 ml (1:1000) SC, IM or IV. When patient undergoes hypovolemic shock, then epinephrine is administered but not alone. It is given along with other fluids like plasma expander (Haemacel) to recover the fluid loss. When patient undergoes severe asthmatic attack, epinephrine is also administered as an emergency to relieve bronchoconstriction.

Dextrose 50% or Glucagon:

They are given parenterally if; diabetic patient undergoes severe hypoglycaemic attack in which the patient may go into syncope.

Corticosteroids:

Hydrocortisone (Solu-cortef)

Methylprednisone (Solu-medrol)

Dexamethasone (Decadron)

In case of severe asthma Solu-cortef, which has an acute onset of action, is administered for immediate relief of bronchoconstriction.

Hydrocortisone Na succinate in a dose of 200 mg IV is given.

In case of allergic reaction involving respiratory system and/ or cardiovascular system, Solu-cortef or Decadron is administered parenterally.

Morphine Sulphate:

It is an opioid, use to relieve severe pain like chest pain due to MI.

Morphine sulphate in a dose of 2 mg is administered IV or SC until the relief of severe chest pain.

Diazepam or Midazolam:

They are anticonvulsant drugs given in status epilepticus. When in dental office patient suffer an attack of seizures, Diazepam 5 mg/min IV is given upto the dose of 10 mg. Alternatively, if no diazepam is available then Midazolam 3 mg/min is administered IV or IM upto 6 mg.

Another alternative is Lorazepam 4 mg given IV at the rate of 2 mg/minute.

If the seizure does not stop with diazepam or Lorazepam then patient is shifted to medical emergency where **phenytoin** is given in a dose of 15 mg/kg IV diluted with 0.9% normal saline at the rate less than 50mg/minute.

Thiamine 250 mg (vitamin B1) may also be given IV, if patient is suspected with poor nutrition or alcohol abuse.

INHALATIONAL DRUGS [8]

Salbutamol, Metaproterenol, or Terbutaline:

These are bronchodilator drugs used for an attack of asthma in an inhaler form. Nebulized Salbutamol 5 mg or terbutaline 10 mg is administered.

Patient with history of asthma should keep these inhalers in their pocket or be made available by dentist in his office whilst performing dental procedure.

Aromatic ammonia:

It is a respiratory stimulant and is used in dental office. If the patient is about to fall into syncope due to anxiety this spirit ammonia is inhaled via nose.

APPENDIX I

PREGNANCY CATEGORIES:

The pregnancy category of pharmaceutical agent is an assessment of the risk of fetal injury due to the pharmaceutical, if it is used by the mother during pregnancy. It doesn't confer any risk in the breast milk.

Pregnancy Category A: (Generally considered safe)

The pregnancy category of pharmaceutical agent is an assessment of the risk of fetal injury due to the pharmaceutical, If it is used by the mother during pregnancy. It does not confer any risk in the breast milk.

Pregnancy Category B: (caution advised)

Animal reproduction studies have failed to demonstrate a risk to the fetus and there are no adequate and well-controlled studies in pregnant women OR animal studies which have shown an adverse effect, but adequate and well-controlled studies in pregnant women have failed to demonstrate a risk to the fetus in any trimester.

Pregnancy Category C: (weigh risk and benefit)

Animal reproduction studies have shown an adverse effect on the fetus and there are no adequate and well-controlled studies in humans, but potential benefits may warrant use of the drug in pregnant women despite potential risks.

Pregnancy Category D: (weigh risk and benefit)

There is positive evidence of human fetal risk based on adverse reaction data from investigational or marketing experience or studies in humans, but potential benefits may warrant use of the drug in pregnant women despite potential risks.

Pregnancy Category X: (contraindicated)

Studies in animals or humans have demonstrated fetal abnormalities and/or there is positive evidence of human fetal risk based on adverse reaction data from investigational or marketing experience, and the risks involved in use of drug in pregnant women clearly outweigh potential benefits. [2]

APPENDIX II

CALCULATION OF MAXIMUM DOSAGES AND NUMBER OF CARTRIDGES OF LOCAL ANAESTHETICS:

1. **Lidocaine:**

   Lidocaine 2%, without vasoconstrictor.

   MRD (maximum recommended dose) 4.4 mg/kg

   1 cartridge = 1.8ml (available in Pakistan)

   Lidocaine 2% = 20mg/ml

   So, Lidocaine 2% per cartridge = 20 x 1.8 = 36mg/cartridge

   For Example for 70 kg person, the, MRD will be calculated as;

   4.4mg/kg = 300 mg = 300 / 36 = 8.33 cartridges (8 cartridges)

   So, maximum of 8 cartridges can be given to this person.

2. **Lidocaine with vasoconstrictor:**

   MRD (maximum recommended dose) 6.6mg/kg = 500mg

   1 cartridge = 1.8 ml

   Lidocaine 2% with vasoconstrictor = 20mg/ml

   So, Lidocaine 2% per cartridge = 36 mg/ cartridge

   So, MRD 500 mg = 500 / 36 = 13.88 cartridges (14 cartridges)

   Therefore maximum of 14 cartridges can be given to a healthy individual weighing 70 kg, but this time vasoconstrictor is added.

3. Bupivacaine with vasoconstrictor:

MRD (maximum recommended dose) 1.3 mg/kg = 90 mg

1 cartridge = 1.8 ml

Bupivacaine 0.5 % with vasoconstrictor = 5mg/ml

So, Bupivacaine 0.5% per 1.8ml cartridge = 5 x 1.8 = 9mg/ cartridge

So, MRD 90 mg = 90 / 9 = 10 cartridges

Therefore maximum of 10 cartridges of Bupivacaine 0.5% can be administered to a healthy individual. [5]

APPENDIX III

Prophylactic Regimens for Dental, Respiratory tract and Oesophageal procedures: [5]

SITUATION	AGENTS	REGIMEN
Standard General prophylaxis	Amoxicillin	Adults: 2 g; Children 50mg/kg orally 1hour prior to procedure
Unable to take oral medications	Ampicillin	Adults: 2 g IM or IV; Children 50mg/kg IM or IV within 30 minutes before procedure
Allergic to penicillin	Clindamycin OR	Adults:600mg; Children 20mg/kg orally 1 hour prior to procedure
	Cephalexin or Cephadroxil	Adults:2 g; Children 50mg/kg orally 1 hour prior to procedure
	OR Azithromycin Or Clarithromycin	Adults: 500mg; Children 15mg/kg orally 1 hour prior to procedure

Allergic to penicillin and unable to take oral medications	Clindamycin OR	Adults: 600mg; Children 20mg/kg IV within 30 minutes prior to procedure
	Cefazolin	Adults: 1g; Children 25mg/kg IM or IV within 30 minutes prior to procedure

APPENDIX IV

Commonly used mouth washes:

Agents	Proprietary names	Actions	Characteristics
Chlorhexidine	Peridex, PerioGuard	Inhibits plaque gingivitis	Unwanted effects include; altered taste sensation, extrinsic staining and supragingival calculas formation
Stannous flouride	Gel-kam, Gum care, Meridol	Inhibits plaque ginigivitis	ADA approved only for anticarious properties
Phenolic oil compound	Listerine	Inhibits plaque gingivitis	Contains alcohol content of 27%
Triclosan (Bis-phenol)	Total	Inhibits plaque gingivitis	—
Cetylpyridinium Chloride	Scope, Cepacol	Inhibits plaque	—

REFERENCES

1. RANG AND DALE'S Pharmacology, seventh Edition
2. Lippincott's ILLUSTRATED Reviews Pharmacology, 4th Edition
3. Betram G. Katzung Basic and Clinical Pharmacology, seventh Edition
4. CARRANZA'S CLINICAL PERIODONTOLOGY, Tenth Edition
5. Handbook of LOCAL ANESTHESIA, STANLEY F. MALAMED, FIFTH Edition
6. Oral pathology J.V. Soames and J.C.Southam, Fourth Edition
7. CAWSON'S Essentials of ORAL PATHOLOGY AND ORAL MEDICINE, Eighth Edition
8. CONTEMPORARY Oral and Maxillofacial Surgery James R. Hupp, Edward Ellis III, Myron R. Tucker, 5th Edition
9. KUMAR & CLARK'S CLINICAL MEDICINE, Seventh Edition
10. Delmar's Dental Drug Reference
11. Endodontics Principles and Practice Mahmoud Torabinejad, 4th Edition

www.ingramcontent.com/pod-product-compliance
Lightning Source LLC
Chambersburg PA
CBHW031832170526
45157CB00001B/276